On Being a Pharmacist

On Being a Pharmacist
True Stories by Pharmacists

Compiled and Edited by

Joanna Maudlin Pangilinan, PharmD, BCOP
Pharmacist
Comprehensive Cancer Center
University of Michigan Health System
Ann Arbor, Michigan

J. Aubrey Waddell, PharmD, FAPhA, BCOP
Associate Professor of Clinical Pharmacy
College of Pharmacy
University of Tennessee Health Science Center
Knoxville, Tennessee

Oncology Pharmacist
Blount Memorial Hospital
Maryville, Tennessee

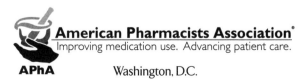

American Pharmacists Association®
Improving medication use. Advancing patient care.
APhA   Washington, D.C.

Acquiring Editor: Sandra J. Cannon
Project Manager: Dean Trackman
Editor: Kathleen A. Savory
Proofreader: Shelly Elliott
Book Design and Layout: Michele A. Danoff, Graphics by Design
Cover Design: Richard Muringer, APhA Creative Services

APhA was founded in 1852 as the American Pharmaceutical Association.

To comment on this book via e-mail, send your message to the publisher at
aphabooks@aphanet.org.

Library of Congress Cataloging-in-Publication Data

On being a pharmacist : true stories by pharmacists / compiled and edited by
Joanna Maudlin Pangilinan, J. Aubrey Waddell.
    p. ; cm.
Includes bibliographical references.
ISBN 978-1-58212-133-8 (alk. paper)
1. Pharmacy. 2. Pharmacists. 3. Pharmacy—Anecdotes. I. Pangilinan,
Joanna Maudlin. II. Waddell, J. Aubrey. III. American Pharmacists Association.
[DNLM: 1. Pharmacists—Personal Narratives. 2. Professional Role—Personal
Narratives. 3. Professional-Patient Relations—Personal Narratives. QV 21 O58 2010]
RS122.5.O5 2010
615'.1—dc22
                                    2009052216

How to Order This Book

Online: www.pharmacist.com/shop_apha
By phone: 800-878-0729 (770-280-0085 from outside the United States)
VISA®, MasterCard®, and American Express® cards accepted.

To my parents, Tom and Roberta,
who gave me my prescription.

To my husband, Jun, and daughters Caroline and Carmen,
who helped me realize my Sig.

—*Joanna Maudlin Pangilinan*

To Dominic, who made me into a pharmacist,
whether or not he wishes to admit to it.

To Dad, the great storyteller of the Waddell clan.

To Debbie, who stole my heart in a drugstore 34 years ago.

To Alex and Austin, joga bonito!

—*J. Aubrey Waddell*

Contents

Contents

Chapter 4 • On Day-to-Day Life

Chapter 5 • On Military Service

Chapter 6 • On Innovative Service

Chapter 7 • On Gifts and Giving

Chapter 8 • On Patient Encounters

Chapter 9 • On Humorous Situations

Chapter 10 • On Ethical Situations

Chapter 11 • On Challenging Situations

Chapter 12 • On Death and Dying

Chapter 13 • On Christmastime

Chapter 14 • On Lessons Learned

Contents

Foreword

I am pleased to share with the readers of *On Being a Pharmacist: True Stories by Pharmacists* two important personal experiences that shaped my vision for pharmacy. The anecdotes, which I included in my Remington Honor Medal speech in April 2009, follow.

The first experience occurred when I was a resident at the Hospital of the University of Pennsylvania; we called it HUP. I was asked to participate on the chief of medicine's patient-care team. We had a patient who had chest pain, and the diagnosis was narrowed down to either an acute myocardial infarction (MI) or a dissecting aortic aneurysm. One of the critical pieces of information that I was asked to provide was whether the patient was hypertensive. I had to do this by checking his medications. The bottle was not labeled, it contained many unidentified medications, the patient's pharmacy was closed, and there was just not enough time to sort through the mess. The team made the decision to treat the patient for an acute MI with standard anticoagulation. Unfortunately, the patient had a dissecting aortic aneurysm and died in part because of the treatment.

Everyone was upset, but I was devastated. Here, during my first real opportunity as a team member, I had little to offer. The chief of medicine sought me out to reassure me that he was responsible and to encourage me to stay the course. This episode rocked my world. I realized that I was unprepared to make a contribution to the patient-care conversations with my medical colleagues. I did not have pathophysiology, therapeutic courses, or clerkship experiences in my education. I went back on rounds. However, I also resolved that our profession's education had to change.

I soon found that I was not alone in this resolution—many colleagues at other colleges of pharmacy had the same dedication to improving pharmacy education. As a result, pharmacists today have the analytical, clinical, and communication skills to better contribute to patient care.

The second experience occurred when I was a patient having back surgery at Johns Hopkins Hospital just this past year. The nurses and physicians were incredibly gifted and dedicated. Yet, it was my pharmacist who helped me the most. He was directly involved in the provision of my care and helped me understand today's remarkably complicated treatments—and what pharmacy's promised land will be like.

By sharing significant professional experiences, pharmacists can help one another recognize their true calling and help the profession more fully realize its potential.

John A. Gans
February 2010

Preface

Pharmacists are amazingly underrepresented in plays, novels, short stories, movies, and television shows, especially when one considers that more than 250,000 pharmacists are in practice today in the United States alone and untold millions have practiced throughout history. One can quickly identify physician and nurse characters in popular drama, but pharmacists are all but invisible. Were it not for the flawed but redeemed Mr. Gower in *It's a Wonderful Life*, nice guy Murphy in *Murphy's Romance*, heroic Tom Craig in *In Old California*, evil George on *Desperate Housewives*, trailblazing Miss Ellie on *The Andy Griffith Show*, and just a few others, pharmacists would be completely missing from the big and small screens.

Perhaps some of that is our own fault. Perhaps we are too caught up in the "perfection is the only standard" nature of the profession to pursue the literary side of what we do. Maybe the people drawn to pharmacy are science, math, and business types who don't see the "story" in what happens to them in a typical day of practice. Could it be that pharmacists are just naturally uninteresting people?

We think not. We are two people who had never met—one in Tennessee and the other in Michigan. We had long thought that pharmacy was full of good storytellers and good stories. At about the same time, we both approached the American Pharmacists Association (APhA) with the idea for a book of true stories about pharmacy practice, told by real pharmacists. Our idea was approved, and we started sending out the word in any way we could think of: e-mails to state pharmacy associations, e-mails to military pharmacy leaders, an open letter in *Pharmacy Today*, a recurring ad in APhA's periodic e-mail newsletter, calls to our many friends and acquaintances in the profession, and podium announcements at statewide continuing education meetings and the APhA Federal Forum. Sometimes, we just asked pharmacists who were complete strangers for stories. And the stories came. Some of them surprised us with their historic importance, some made us laugh, some made us think, and some were just plain unique. In this Internet age, it didn't take too long until we received stories that had to be translated from a foreign language.

We have enjoyed receiving and reading these stories and getting to know a little about the authors. Our hope is that this little book will make others like us decide to get out a pen and paper (or a computer) and write down that meaningful or funny or sad event that happened in a community pharmacy, in a hospital pharmacy, in a compounding pharmacy, in a school of pharmacy, in the military, in the pharmaceutical industry, in an association—in any setting where any kind of pharmacy is practiced. We hope that these stories are then told: shared with students, included in professional presentations, published in our professional journals, or sent to us for a future edition of this book.

Pharmacy has come so far professionally, economically, educationally, and clinically. It's time to take the next step and have the profession become part of society's literary consciousness, not as an occasional visitor but as a permanent, helpful, professional friend.

J. Aubrey Waddell
Joanna Maudlin Pangilinan

Acknowledgments

This book would not have been possible without the American Pharmacists Association, which gave us an opportunity to showcase the thoughts and experiences of pharmacists from around the world. Thank you APhA Books and Electronic Products Department, especially Sandy Cannon and Julian Graubart, for your support and guidance.

This book would also not have been possible without the support of our fellow pharmacists. Whether you sent us a story or helped pass around word of our project, we thank you for helping us with this book. This book is by you, about you, and for you.

Contributors

Jane McKimens Adams, MS, RPh
Pharmacy Clinical Coordinator
Medication Safety
St. Luke's Episcopal Hospital
Houston, Texas

Anita Airee, PharmD
Assistant Professor of Clinical Pharmacy
College of Pharmacy
University of Tennessee Health
  Science Center
Knoxville, Tennessee

Nancy A. Alvarez, PharmD, BCPS, FAPhA
Director, Medical Information
Medical Affairs Department
Endo Pharmaceuticals, Inc.
Chadds Ford, Pennsylvania

Gary R. Anderson, RPh
Director of Pharmacy
Northfield Hospital
Northfield, Minnesota

John Backus, PharmD
Fort Myers, Florida

Rosalie Bader, BSP
Canada Safeway
Moose Jaw, Saskatchewan, Canada

Luigi Barlassina, MPharm Chemistry
Pharmacist Manager
Regional Late-Night Pharmacy
Cork, Ireland

Paul R. Bergeron II, RPh
Retail Community Pharmacist
Lake Monticello, Virginia

Janet Bradshaw, BSP
Dysart, Saskatchewan, Canada

Jef Bratberg, PharmD, BCPS
Clinical Associate Professor, Pharmacy
  Practice
University of Rhode Island
Kingston, Rhode Island
Assistant Professor, Medicine (Clinical)
Brown University
Providence, Rhode Island
Infectious Diseases Specialist
Roger Williams Medical Center
Providence, Rhode Island

Peter A. Chyka, PharmD
Professor and Executive Associate Dean
College of Pharmacy
University of Tennessee Health
  Science Center
Knoxville, Tennessee

Sharon Connor, PharmD
Assistant Professor
University of Pittsburgh School of
  Pharmacy
Pittsburgh, Pennsylvania

Kathleen J. Cross, PharmD
Christus St. John Hospital
Nassau Bay, Texas

Steve Cummings, RPh
Director of Pharmacy Services
Marsh Drugs, LLC
Indianapolis, Indiana

Robert DeChristoforo, MS, FASHP
Captain, U.S. Public Health Service (Ret.)
Chief, Pharmacy Department
Clinical Center
National Institutes of Health
Bethesda, Maryland

Michael P. Dunphy, RPh, MS
Director, Continuing Education
South Carolina College of Pharmacy
Columbia, South Carolina

Ashley W. Ellis, PharmD
Clinical Assistant Professor, Pharmacy
  Practice
University of Mississippi School of
  Pharmacy
University, Mississippi

Heather Eppert, PharmD, BCPS
Assistant Professor of Clinical Pharmacy
College of Pharmacy
University of Tennessee Health
  Science Center
Knoxville, Tennessee
Clinical Specialist, Emergency Medicine
Blount Memorial Hospital
Maryville, Tennessee

Mollie Kidorf Fisch, RPh, MS
Teaneck, New Jersey

Eric Foss, RPh
CHN Pharmacy
Wautoma, Wisconsin

Andrea S. Franks, PharmD, BCPS
Associate Professor of Clinical Pharmacy
Director of Education
College of Pharmacy
University of Tennessee Health
  Science Center
Knoxville, Tennessee

Patrick Garman, PharmD, PhD
Lieutenant Colonel, U.S. Army

Mark Garofoli, PharmD, MBA

Christa M. George, PharmD, BCPS, CDE
Assistant Professor of Clinical Pharmacy
College of Pharmacy
University of Tennessee Health
  Science Center
Memphis, Tennessee

Kathryn L. Hahn, PharmD, DAAPM
Affiliate Faculty
Oregon State University College of
  Pharmacy
Clinical Instructor
Pacific University College of Pharmacy
Chair
Oregon Pain Management Commission
State Action Leader
American Pain Foundation
Pharmacy Manager
Bi-Mart Corp.
Springfield, Oregon

Lynn Harrelson, BPharm, FASCP
Senior Care Pharmacist
President
Senior Pharmacy Solutions
Louisville, Kentucky

W. Mike Heath, RPh, MBA
Colonel, U.S. Army (Ret.)
Martinez, Georgia

Mary Herbert, MS, MPH
Clinical Director
Program for Health Care to Underserved
  Populations
Division of General Internal Medicine
University of Pittsburgh
Pittsburgh, Pennsylvania

William O. Hiner Jr., MS, RPh
Colonel, U.S. Army (Ret.)
Southampton, Pennsylvania

Darrell Hulisz, PharmD
Associate Professor, Family Medicine
Case Western Reserve University School
  of Medicine
Associate Clinical Professor, Pharmacy
  Practice
Ohio Northern University College of
  Pharmacy
Cleveland, Ohio

Jason Hutchens, PharmD
Clinical Pharmacy Specialist
Blount Memorial Hospital
Maryville, Tennessee

Heather J. Johnson, PharmD, BCPS
Assistant Professor, Pharmacy and
  Therapeutics
University of Pittsburgh School of
  Pharmacy
Clinical Pharmacist, Transplant ICU
University of Pittsburgh Medical Center
Pittsburgh, Pennsylvania

Mike Johnson, RPh
Assistant Director, Pharmacy
Blount Memorial Hospital
Maryville, Tennessee

**Julian Judge, MPSI, BSc(Pharm),
  Dip Grad Psych**
Proprietor
Old Bawn Pharmacy
Dublin, Ireland

Rosalyn C. King, PharmD, MPH
Program Manager (Ret.)
Office of International Programs
Howard University Continuing
  Education
Washington, D.C.

**Koninklijke Nederlandse Maatschappij
  ter bevordering der Pharmacie**
The Koninklijke Nederlandse
Maatschappij ter bevordering der
Pharmacie (Royal Dutch Association
for the Advancement of Pharmacy)
is the umbrella organization in the
Netherlands for professional pharmacists
and pharmacy in general. It promotes
both the interests of its members and the
interests of the pharmaceutical sector.

Robert A. Lucas, PharmD
Blount Memorial Hospital
Maryville, Tennessee

Robert A. Lytle, RPh
Lytle Pharmacy
Rochester, Michigan

Sarah T. Melton, PharmD, BCPP, CGP
Director, Addiction Outreach
Associate Professor, Pharmacy Practice
Appalachian College of Pharmacy
Oakwood, Virginia

Aaron P. Middlekauff, PharmD
Lieutenant Commander, U.S. Public
  Health Service
Alaska Native Medical Center
Anchorage, Alaska

Mary Ann Mobilian, PharmD candidate
University of Florida
Jacksonville, Florida

Fintan Moore, BSc(Pharm)
Green Park Pharmacy
Dublin, Ireland

Nancy L. Mueller, RPh
Comprehensive Cancer Center
University of Michigan Health System
Ann Arbor, Michigan

Stephen L. Murley, RPh
Boerne, Texas

Martin Niedelman, BPharm
Roslyn, New York

Olafur Olafsson, MSc Pharm
AstraZeneca
Reykjavik, Iceland

Fred J. Pane, BPharm
Senior Director, Pharmacy Affairs
Premier, Inc.
Charlotte, North Carolina

Joanna Maudlin Pangilinan, PharmD, BCOP
Comprehensive Cancer Center
University of Michigan Health System
Ann Arbor, Michigan

Keith Patterson, PharmD
Emergency Room Pharmacist
Northside Hospital–Forsyth
Cumming, Georgia

Doreen Pon, PharmD, BCOP
Assistant Professor, Pharmacy Practice
  and Administration
Western University of Health Sciences
Pomona, California
Faculty in Residence
City of Hope National Medical Center
Duarte, California

Charles D. Ponte, PharmD, CDE, BCPS, BC-ADM, FASHP, FCCP, FAPhA
Professor, Clinical Pharmacy and Family
  Medicine
Robert C. Byrd Health Sciences Center
West Virginia University Schools of
  Pharmacy and Medicine
Morgantown, West Virginia

Kelly Procailo, PharmD
Comprehensive Cancer Center
University of Michigan Health System
Ann Arbor, Michigan

David K. Records, BPharm
Associate Consultant–Regulatory
Lilly Research Laboratories Regulatory
  Affairs
Global Operations Labeling Department
Eli Lilly and Company
Indianapolis, Indiana

L. Douglas Ried, PhD
Dean
Southwestern Oklahoma State
 University
Weatherford, Oklahoma

Donald Rolls, RPh
Comprehensive Cancer Center
University of Michigan Health System
Ann Arbor, Michigan

Lisa M. Scholz, PharmD, MBA
Senior Director
HRSA Pharmacy Services Support Center
American Pharmacists Association
Washington, D.C.

Michael J. Schuh, PharmD, MBA
Assistant Professor, Pharmacy
Mayo College of Medicine
Ambulatory Pharmacist
Mayo Clinic
Jacksonville, Florida

Mary Shue, RPh
University of Michigan Health System
Ann Arbor, Michigan

Nancy Brady Smith, RPh,
 CDM-Diabetes
Walgreens
Huron, Ohio

Pamela Stewart-Kuhn, RPh, MPA, CGP
Captain, U.S. Public Health Service
Chief, Health Services Division
U.S. Coast Guard Aviation Training
 Center
Mobile, Alabama

Jessica Stovel, Hon BSc, BScPhm
Pediatric Pharmacist
Victoria Hospital
London Health Sciences Centre
London, Ontario, Canada

Giorgio Tosolini
Farmacista Territoriale
Italy

J. Aubrey Waddell, PharmD, FAPhA,
 BCOP
Associate Professor of Clinical Pharmacy
College of Pharmacy
University of Tennessee Health
 Science Center
Knoxville, Tennessee
Oncology Pharmacist
Blount Memorial Hospital
Maryville, Tennessee

Keith A. Wagner, PharmD
Lieutenant Colonel, U.S. Army

William R. Wills, RPh, FIACP
Grandpa's Compounding Pharmacy
Placerville, California

Warren D. Winston, RPh
RPh on the Go
Pittsfield, Illinois

Michelle Zingone, PharmD, BCPS
Assistant Professor of Clinical Pharmacy
College of Pharmacy
University of Tennessee Health
 Science Center
Knoxville, Tennessee

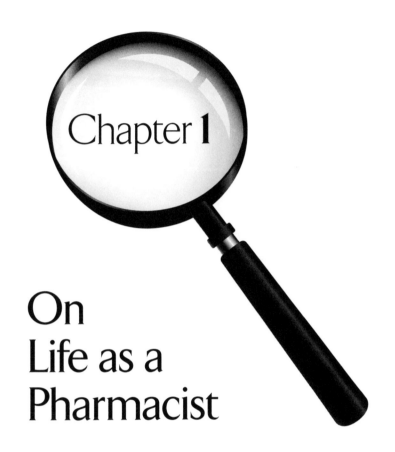

Chapter 1

On Life as a Pharmacist

Every day, in every way,
I'm getting better.

—**Émile Ćoue,** *French*
pharmacist and psychologist

It Is What You Make It

Robert A. Lytle, RPh

My guess is that this book will be read mostly by pharmacists and the families of those who contribute articles to it. What it certainly will do is give practicing pharmacists a rare chance to express in print the inside life of what we do every day—to describe at length the gratifying experiences that keep us going in the face of all the annoyances: the voice-activated messages, inconsiderate receptionists, and last-minute customers.

What I would like to tell you is how and why I became a pharmacist.

When I was 7 years old, my mother was stricken with a paralyzing form of rheumatoid arthritis. Our corner drugstore was only a couple of blocks from our house. It often was my job to fetch mom's medication. Mr. B was the pharmacist and owner. He was also highly respected by everyone, extremely active in the community, and even elected as our district's representative in the state house of representatives. He was a big deal.

As you may know, kids are great observers. I was no exception. I noticed quickly that every time I walked into Mr. B's drugstore, he greeted me with "Hey, Bobby, how was school today?" or "How's your mom, Bobby?" I noticed that he also greeted everyone else by name, and by doing so, he made all of us feel special. And isn't feeling special a part of helping sick people get better? Although that alone didn't directly help my mom, it did make *me* feel better about coming to his drugstore as my role in helping her.

All right, maybe he did it for his own good. After all, fast, friendly service is not just a buzz phrase; it's good business to let your customers know that their trade is appreciated. But, I think that line of reasoning is too cynical. Anyone who spends as much time as pharmacists do in one place finds that work is so much more enjoyable if the customers are also friends. And what better way to make friends than to do something for others, whether it is going the extra mile by contacting a doctor, getting the best price on a prescription, or simply greeting customers by their first names.

I was in about the eighth grade when I decided that I wanted to be like Mr. B—to be a pharmacist and have a store in my own town. I checked out what was required to become a pharmacist. Throughout my high school years, I took courses that led to that end. I went to pharmacy school; got married along the way; graduated; and, with my wife, began to look for a town where I could set up shop and be like Mr. B.

I landed in Rochester, Michigan, a small town that both my wife and I loved. I got a job with a large national chain and worked there for 7 years, all the while looking for a storefront that I could lease to start my own store. One day, the most wonderful, independently owned, downtown drugstore—one that had been on the busiest corner of town for more than 150 years—became available. With the financial help of a very understanding family, I jumped in, feet first, and bought it. Since then, I have done everything I could to be like Mr. B, the pharmacist I always hoped to be.

I soon found that knowing my customers' names was just the tip of the iceberg. To compete with my former chain store and all the other drugstores in the area, I had to get involved in community affairs. That included church, school, service clubs, local politics, and sports. I had to win the respect of the townspeople to attract their business. Even then, once I had earned their loyalty, I was always at risk of losing them to forced mail-order plans, new competition, or dozens of other factors. It is and has been a constant battle.

I've been told it's a minor miracle that an independent pharmacist still survives in an era of mail-order pressure and chain-store domination. Yet, I compete with their enormous advertising budgets, vast parking lots, and carload purchasing power by carving a niche with personal service, reasonable pricing, and community service. Even in the depths of the current challenging economic times, I have been able to thrive while watching the chain stores, one right after the next, come and go.

To close, I emphasize this: People will, given the opportunity, patronize a store that provides reasonably priced goods, fast service, and a cheerful greeting, one such as I received from Mr. B 50-some years ago when he smiled at me and said, "Hi, Bobby, how's your mom?" ●

A Pharmacist's Almanac

Mollie Kidorf Fisch, RPh, MS

I was born into pharmacy, and it has been very good to me. Now I am retired but maintain my New Jersey license as a point of pride—and just in case!

My father was a graduate of Temple University, class of 1922, and owned a corner drugstore in a Philadelphia neighborhood. He started as a young fellow, and his very distinguished looking, white-haired father, who didn't know a thing about medication, liked to help out in the front of the store. Folks who came in preferred to speak with the "old Doc" in those days, so they would tell my grandfather what troubled them. He would "consult" with my dad, who would advise the customers what to take for their ailments, and everyone was happy. Before long, my dad became "Doc" in his own right and gained the full trust of the entire neighborhood. He always knew his boundaries, helping people to the best of his ability and sending them to a physician when needed. He never thought of charging a consulting fee. He just gave of himself freely and always with a smile.

Living upstairs from the store meant that my brother and I spent a lot of time working alongside our parents—my mother also worked in the drugstore. For me, that was always interesting and fun, and I often traded off hours with my brother, who was less enamored of the experience.

When I was 16 years old and still in high school, I applied for my apprenticeship papers, which was the way one began in pharmacy in the early 1950s. So, by the time I had graduated from Temple University College of Pharmacy in 1956, one of 10 women in a class of 110 and the last year of the 4-year program, I had only another month or so of internship. I had no trouble passing my boards in Pennsylvania, New York, and New Jersey. We did a lot of compounding in those days, and I aced all the practical exams on capsules, powders, ointments, and handmade suppositories.

I started out working in stores and then moved on to the hospital environment. When I got married and moved to New Jersey, I worked in the local Catholic hospital, which also had a 3-year school of nursing and a school of practical nursing. In addition to working as a staff pharmacist, I was soon enlisted to teach pharmacology to the nursing students. I also taught in-service classes for nurses, particularly in the hemodialysis unit and the respiratory therapy area, on new or specialized medications. That was a perfect solution to my desire to stay active professionally while raising a family. When my two children were small, I focused on the teaching, with just a few hours a week as a staff pharmacist. As the children got older and less dependent, my hours in the pharmacy increased.

In my 40s, my husband encouraged me to return to school for a master's degree in pharmacy, because he said, "I am tired of hearing you come home from continuing education lectures saying that you could have taught the material better than the instructor. Go get an advanced degree!" After 2 years of night classes at Long Island University's (LIU's) Arnold & Marie Schwartz College of Pharmacy and Health Sciences, I earned my degree, with a specialization in drug information. And just by chance, I looked in the newspaper and saw a posting for a position in the pharmaceutical industry that was right up my alley!

After 19 years in the hospital, I spent 20 years in industry, working in the medical services department of the international marketing division of a pharmaceutical company. I moved from medical writer and editor to manager, and eventually to director of international labeling in the same company. Every day was an adventure in learning something new.

My department prepared package inserts for the clinician and the patient and negotiated these inserts through regulatory affairs in various countries worldwide. I initiated an industry rotation, and students from Rutgers College of Pharmacy came through our department under my preceptorship. As adjunct professor at LIU, I taught a course in medical writing for the pharmaceutical industry. When I retired from my full-time job in 2004, I was asked to become a consultant for another large company in its U.S. division. Additionally, throughout my career, I have enjoyed presenting programs in local schools on the proper use of medication and on pharmacy as a career.

I have seen so many changes in the field of pharmacy, both technological and sociological. The technological advances have been tremendous, and the advances sociologically are just as great. When I started, the field was male dominated. Now, many bright women have chosen pharmacy as a career, and much more diversity is accepted.

At the beginning of my career, I had three strikes against me: I was young, female, and an Orthodox Jew who could not work on Saturdays or Jewish holidays. It was not easy to get that first job, but once I did get hired, I earned the respect of my colleagues. The youthful part was handled by nature. The other two became less important to my bosses as society changed. The end result was a wonderful career, allowing me to take advantage of many unusual opportunities and work with interesting people worldwide.

My experience shows just how varied and interesting the field of pharmacy has been—and remains. So many different opportunities and experiences are available if you are open to them. How was I so fortunate? The following attitudes helped me a great deal to work with whatever opportunities and challenges life sent my way:

○ Keep positive: Find the upside to any job. (I never met a job in pharmacy that I did not like in some way.)
○ Keep learning: Seek educational opportunities throughout your life.
○ Keep growing: Strive for both professional and personal development.
○ Keep trying: Remember that if one thing doesn't work out, something else will.
○ Keep mentoring: Help those coming up in the field—young people are our future. ●

The Phainting Pharmacist

Kelly Procailo, PharmD

I chose pharmacy because I know I get queasy.
I soon found out, it just isn't that easy.
I thought it would be the perfect career.
Little did I know, there was still much to fear!

All gowned up, sporting my crocs,
To the OR I went to help out the docs.
All they asked of me was to do a heparin flush.
Moments later, I lay on the floor—instant mush!
Yes, I, a pharmacist, became an ER patient.
Safer for me to work in the pharmacy located in the basement!

The life of trauma/burn
Became quite the concern.
Knowing what I would see day to day rounding
Sent my heart a-pounding.
Reviewing a patient chart outside the room,
Everyone turned once they heard the "boom."
Boy, this fainting was starting to take its toll,
Making me want to disappear into a hole!

Oh, don't worry, that wasn't the last episode.
It is truly unpredictable when the next time I may fold.
Not dwelling on the past, looking forward to tomorrow,
The strength and support of others, I can borrow.
There is always a place in the pharmacy world for me, I know.
All I need to do is take a deep breath and go with the flow! ●

Life as a Small-Town Pharmacist

Eric Foss, RPh

I began as a pharmacist in a small rural town, where I had recently moved. It was, and is, a pleasant town of about 5,000 people in the gently rolling woods and farmland of central Wisconsin. As such, I found that patients got to know me well—more so than is typical of even frequent patients in a larger city, such as where I had interned.

Shortly after I started, I was buying gas and went in to pay. The lady behind the counter was looking at me quizzically as I paid and then suddenly smiled and burst out, "Oh, I know who you are. You're my favorite pharmacist!" This was my introduction to being, as I call it, "almost famous."

Some time after that, I had reason to call one of my patients at home about her prescription. This was in the days before caller ID. The phone rang, and an obviously very young boy answered. Without bothering to identify myself because of the child's young age, I asked, "Could I speak to Mrs. Jones please?"

I heard a thud as the child put down the phone, and then I heard the boy call out to his mother in a very loud voice, "Mommm, it's the pharmaciiiist!" I was amazed to think that this child knew who I was just by my voice.

Thus began a litany of patient interactions, much of it outside of work. One thing I have always enjoyed is that I actually hear back from my patients about information we have discussed or recommendations I have made. Even weeks later, a patient might walk up to the counter with a "Hey, thanks! That cream you told me to get for my poison ivy really worked." Or an "I finally quit coughing and was able to sleep."

One day, a lady came into the pharmacy. She looked familiar, but I didn't immediately recognize her. She had been in a few weeks before to ask me what to do about a swollen leg. Now, obviously I'm not a doctor, but having just one leg swollen instead of two sent off little alarm bells in my head. Trying not to be too distressing, I very firmly told her that she should go see her doctor immediately. It turns out that she took my advice and was admitted to the hospital with deep venous thrombosis.

Standing at the counter now, she had a simple thank you for me, saying, "My doctor told me to tell you that you saved my life." I was speechless for a second and then told her that I was glad she was now doing well and that I was just doing my job, but she was very welcome.

Being in a small town, it is common to run into patients outside of work— while out to dinner or in the aisles of the grocery store. Sometimes, it's just a smile and a hello. Other times, it's a 20-minute conversation about life, the weather, local happenings, or, of course, their medicine. Sometimes, when in a hurry, I have wished I could be anonymous and just go about my business, but most days I wouldn't trade being recognized for the world. Is this how Harrison Ford feels when he runs errands?

Amazingly, with the number of people you come to know and the even larger number who know you, you encounter patients in the craziest places, even far away from home. It might be at the mall an hour away, the visitors' center at a favorite vacation spot up north, the rest stop on the way to a college football game, or even farther away than that. Twice I have run into patients while on vacation in Florida, 1,400 miles from home.

A particularly memorable moment was as I was walking along at Disney World. I saw a man, with his elderly mother in a wheelchair, trying to safely maneuver her down a short flight of steps. Seeing him struggle and concerned for her safety, I offered to help him lift her in the chair and carry her down the steps. He hoisted his side, and I mine. As we handily got her down the steps, she looked up at me, and I down at her, and we realized that we knew each other.

She was a frequent and delightful patient whom I knew well. She instantly smiled and began chatting up a storm with me. Her poor son, not knowing who I was or that we knew each other, thought that his mother had lost her mind as she talked to this stranger from out of the blue like she had known him forever. He seemed very relieved to find out that I was, in fact, his mother's pharmacist. She and I laugh about that event to this day.

After living and practicing for a while in a town like this, even though you weren't born here, your many interactions with others eventually make you part of the fabric of the town. Your life becomes intertwined with the lives of everybody else, whether friend, neighbor, acquaintance, or even stranger. Connections exist because you share a common tapestry, woven together by the many different relationships and events that make up life. This realization came to me after one of my son's former baseball coaches told me a story.

As I was coaching first base at a game as best I could, the former coach was in the bleachers talking to one of the new dads in town as they watched their boys play. "Hey," the coach said to the dad, "Do you know who that is?" He was pointing at me. The dad replied that no, he did not. "That guy out there is the biggest drug dealer in town! On top of that, everybody knows it and nobody does anything about it. Even the teachers and cops all know, and he's been doing it for years!"

The dad looked at him, incredulous, and asked, "Why not?"

"Because," the coach said, as he started laughing, "he's a pharmacist."

He and I got a good laugh as he told me how he had pulled the dad's leg, and there it was. Known to almost everybody, even those who are not my patients; that is me, "the pharmacist."

Not that long ago I took another job, just a short distance from my old one. I still live in the same town and run into the same people at the grocery store, but now I work in an even smaller town—2,000 people—a few miles away. I still see some of my old patients at my new pharmacy, but many new ones have been added—new lives, new stories, yet in a way, the same. The stories and faces may vary, but the twinkle in the eye, the knowing nod at the occasional inside joke, the heavy sigh if it's been a bit rough, and the smile as they walk in the door and see "the pharmacist" are unchanged. What better title? "The pharmacist"—a person they have come to know and trust, and share a bit of their lives with.

As part of my new job, I write a little column in the local paper, which includes my picture. I get comments on my articles, or even the picture itself. "Hey, I saw your picture in the paper." Conversation ensues. I discover that one patient goes to a barber who happens to be the man I bought my house from. Another patient sees a doctor I went to college with. An officer in the local sheriff's department is a former pharmacy technician of mine. The retired librarian from my pharmacy school sees my picture in the paper and stops in to say hi.

Many lives all intertwined. That's what it's all about, isn't it? The little difference we can make in our patients' lives, and they in ours, all while being "the pharmacist," and maybe just a little bit more. ●

A Decade in the Life of the "Drug Police," aka the Pharmacist

Lisa M. Scholz, PharmD, MBA

When I became a pharmacist more than 10 years ago, I never thought I would experience the wide array of tragedy, professional enlightenment, and pride that I have had the opportunity to be a part of in this profession. When I started pharmacy, I was 16 years old. I was a motivated high school student in need of cash to buy a car, gas, and insurance. The pharmacist interviewed me and decided she would give me a chance, because I was the first high school applicant to give her a resume. Little did I know how hard I would work for my money: $2.85 an hour! Little did she know that she had begun to shape my professional career as a pharmacist.

Growing up in a household of a public servant, my first instinct was to enter into a profession to help people. I grew up the daughter of a police officer. I am proud of what police officers provide to their community—security, safety, and impartiality. I experienced things most children think exist only in the movies. I went on sting operations, helicopter rides, and police car ride-alongs. When it was time for my psychology project, I hit the streets of Houston, Texas, armed with a video recorder and my dad to find out why teenagers abused drugs and joined gangs.

For me, being a part of the community was important, and helping the community was a must. I continued to pursue community involvement throughout high school and college. Upon graduating from pharmacy school, I was faced with the decision of working in my local community or working for the local government health system. My calling was to the local government.

When I started in the community health center as the pharmacy supervisor, I was given the opportunity by the director of the center, a nurse, to run a pharmacy with 10 staff. The wait time at the pharmacy was 3 hours, and I was tasked with lowering it. I quickly realized that my 5 years of Spanish was invaluable for serving these patients and reducing the wait time.

I was able to speak with the patients, answer questions, and help them learn the importance of taking their medications appropriately. The wait time was lowered to 30 minutes. Additionally, a pharmacy referral system, in which patients with special needs were referred to me, was implemented. My patients were from all walks of life, including some of the most despairing in the nation. Even so, I was given many gifts: food, homemade trinkets, and notes of thanks. The greatest gift though was that my patients taught me how to give back through listening, attentiveness, and empathy. From them, I learned compassion, understanding, and humility.

After years of service and several promotions later, I became director of pharmacy for the health system and faced my biggest challenges when Hurricane Katrina hit New Orleans. I was called the morning of the storm and told that 25,000 patients were showing up at the Astroarena, and we needed to build a pharmacy with the capacity to serve patients who had been deprived of medications for days in just 3 hours! My team pulled together our resources and constructed a makeshift intake pharmacy, pickup zone, and waiting room. The saddest day of my career thus far was watching adult parents ignore their crying children as they sat patiently in a coma-like state, waiting for pain pills, heart medications, and other lifesaving drugs.

I had many other sad days: releasing a pharmacist from work for drug diversion, informing a pharmacist of a fatal error, and deciding to leave Houston for Washington, D.C. However, all too many happy days made up for each of the days of sorrow and tragedy. Those happy days made me realize that my career as a pharmacist could affect peoples' lives across the country. I became involved with the Health Resources and Services Administration (HRSA) Pharmacy Services Support Center at the American Pharmacists Association (APhA) and provided technical assistance to underserved communities across the nation. I also volunteered to be an active member of the Medical Reserve Corps in Houston.

My story has only just begun. I have moved from Texas to Washington, D.C., to become a part of the APhA team. I've married a pharmacist and inherited a stepdaughter and son-in-law, both pharmacists. I have left my legacy in Texas to continue a legacy in our nation's capital. I now have responsibility for the HRSA Pharmacy Services Support Center. I am able to help patients and providers daily as the center works to ensure access to prescription drugs and needed clinical pharmacy services to improve medication use in our nation's most vulnerable populations. Pharmacy has been an important part of my life and will continue to be for decades to come. ●

Amazing Journey

Aaron P. Middlekauff, PharmD

I enlisted in the Air Force right out of high school and found myself being stationed at Misawa Air Base in Japan. As much as I had misgivings about going to Japan, it ended up being a fantastic experience. I took night classes and pursued the Air Force Reserve Officers' Training Corps (ROTC) scholarship. Months came and went, and one morning after working a mid-shift, I came home to a voicemail of a raspy-voiced staff sergeant who announced that I had been accepted into the program. It was a dream come true.

I was able to attend Drake University back home in Iowa because of the opportunity afforded me by the ROTC program. Drake was also where I met my beautiful wife Jane, who was in my pharmacy class. She motivated me to pursue my dream and kept me going through working 20 hours a week, keeping up with the ROTC commitments, and maintaining my grades above the 3.0 grade point necessary to retain my scholarship.

Upon graduation, my wife and I received an assignment to the U.S. Air Force Academy, where we gained valuable experience in the inpatient, outpatient, and clinical arenas. After spending just 2 years there, we were assigned to Elmendorf Air Force Base in Anchorage, Alaska. It was there that I served the final time remaining on my commitment to the Air Force.

Immediately upon discharge, I was elated to be fortunate enough to transfer into the U.S. Public Health Service (PHS). I am currently working for the Alaska Native Medical Center, where I am able to engage in 100 percent patient-oriented care with a focus on putting my clinical skills to work. What a fantastic opportunity to be able to see patients, check labs, discuss treatment modalities, and ensure that the patients have a comprehensive understanding of their medication therapy.

It has been an amazing journey. Who knew when I left for basic training just 1 month after high school graduation that I would one day be sharing this story with you. I look forward to the continued adventures in pharmacy through the opportunities set forth by being a part of PHS. ●

The Casual Pharmacist

Nancy L. Mueller, RPh

Six years after leaving the University of Washington College of Pharmacy and working as a hospital pharmacist, an amazing opportunity presented itself. My husband, Bob, was offered a job in Saudi Arabia with the Arabian American Oil Company (ARAMCO).

Experiencing life in a different culture was something I had enjoyed before. As a Rotary Club exchange student in high school, I learned the language and customs of the Danish people by living and going to school in Denmark. I even had the pleasure of working part time at a Danish pharmacy called Sonderbro Apotek in Kolding on the Jutland Peninsula. Working there was a far cry from the corner drugstore where I had worked in Lakewood, Washington.

Now we were on the cusp of a new adventure! We could only speculate on what awaited us in Dhahran, Saudi Arabia.

We were informed by ARAMCO that I would not be able to work as a pharmacist within the company because the company medical center was not hiring American pharmacists. I thought this would be my time to relax and live a life of leisure: a pleasant prospect, since I had worked most of my life.

Disembarking from the 747 at Dhahran airport was like stepping into the bowels of a blast furnace. Heat radiated from the tarmac in waves, and I truly believed an egg would fry on the pavement. Guards armed with machine guns were in attendance as we made our way from the plane to the terminal. Welcome to Saudi Arabia!

An employee from the department where Bob would be working met us after we cleared customs. Don drove us out to our new home: a single-wide trailer in the middle of a dirt field. This was known as "North Camp." Eventually, we would move "On Camp," which was the official ARAMCO company town of Dhahran, where the housing was more like the condominiums in an American suburb.

Experiencing the culture as a native was not in the cards. We were not encouraged to fraternize with the locals, and it was definitely a man's world. Women were not allowed to drive off camp, and buses were provided for us to go into town to shop in Khobar and at the souks in Dammam. I used my free time to try to learn some Arabic, practice on the piano we acquired in Dhahran, explore the areas I could, and attempt to fit in as a housewife.

Local pharmacies were surprisingly similar to American ones. The big difference was you could walk in, request a medication, and it was sold to you without a prescription. Amazing! The shops in town were pretty much run by Lebanese businessmen with Saudi partners. They all spoke English and were amused with our attempts to speak Arabic.

One day, Bob came home from work with news that Dhahran Medical Center was hiring pharmacists. He told me I could be hired as what ARAMCO called a "casual" employee, because regular employees were not being recruited for pharmacist positions. It appeared that my days as a member of the "out-to-lunch bunch" might be over.

All it took to become an inpatient hospital pharmacist in Saudi Arabia was official notary seals from the U.S. secretary of state on all my diplomas. This took about 30 days, working through the U.S. consulate near Dhahran. I was once again gainfully employed—like it or not.

Dhahran Medical Center was accredited and not dissimilar to the other medical centers I had previously worked in. The difference was the people. I was finally able to gain insight into the lives of Saudi Arabians through interactions with the Saudi techs and pharmacists I worked with. It was a truly amazing experience I could have had only as a pharmacist.

My tenure there lasted about 4 years, until I decided to stay home with my twin son and daughter, who were born in the medical center. I look back fondly on my time there, and I know that it had an impact on the rest of my career and life. ●

From Watts to the World: One Pharmacist's Journey

Rosalyn C. King, PharmD, MPH

It happens every time I pass the corner of 23rd and Constitution Avenue, NW, in Washington, D.C. I wonder about other pharmacists who might have worked in two nearby buildings: the American Pharmacists Association (APhA) headquarters and the U.S. Department of State (DOS). The conjunction of work in these two places was significant in guiding the trajectory of my career as a pharmacist and public health professional.

In 1969, APhA brought me to Washington, D.C., from the Watts Health Clinic in South Central Los Angeles to take a position as assistant director of a U.S. Office of Economic Opportunity (OEO)–funded project called The Delivery of Pharmaceutical Services to Poverty Areas of the United States, joining two other pharmacists. I was the first African American pharmacist professional to be employed at APhA headquarters. In 1980, I joined the Health Office in the Africa Bureau of the U.S. Agency for International Development (USAID), located in the DOS building, as a special consultant and public health adviser on pharmaceuticals.

The content of the work with the OEO project yielded a report whose principles and constructs are emphasized even today in community health clinics, centers, and programs across the United States.[1] However, it is the process of applying a pharmacist's knowledge to a health care system's efficiency as a part of the health care team that sparked my story in pharmacy and many of my later efforts. Indeed, one of the realizations that emerged while on the OEO project was that pharmacists are needed as a concrete factor in achieving the goals of most health care systems. Cain and Khan chronicle the elements of this "new," at that time, concept for the public health community.[2]

After being the only pharmacist in my master of public health program in 1972, the call of public health was compelling. The traditional practices of the profession of pharmacy, my focus since completing my first pharmacy degree, were left behind as my role and activities in public health grew. Serving as the only pharmacist on two teams that evaluated pharmaceutical services in over three dozen community health centers across the United States and becoming active in the American Public Health Association augmented my pharmacy–public health focus from 1972 to 1976. It was this background that led to the request that I join USAID for a period of 5 years (1980–1985), beginning with the Africa Bureau.

USAID was beginning to emphasize primary health care in its health assistance efforts, and often a program's problem point was the management of the drug supply to the programs and patients being served. In my work with the agency, I had the opportunity to evaluate and recommend policy and program changes in some 22 countries of Africa, Asia, Latin America and the Caribbean, and the Near East.

This trajectory continued with 7 years as director of the International Health Institute at Charles R. Drew University of Medicine and Science and over 15 years as a program manager for the Office of International Programs (OIP) at Howard University Continuing Education (HUCE), which included developing the Pharmacists and Continuing Education (PACE) Center. At the 15-year celebration of OIP in February 2008, it was noted that approximately 2,310 middle- to senior-level officials from 27 countries and the United States have had their skills enhanced through the OIP. This included nearly 1,000 pharmacists trained in Romania to focus more on their role as care agents versus managers of distribution, as reported by Dr. Felicia Loghin, dean of the faculty of pharmacy at the University of Medicine and Pharmacy in Cluj, Romania. Dr. Loghin acknowledged the mutual benefit for her university and for the pharmacists of Romania. For this and related efforts, the university's faculty senate voted to award me an honorary professorship in 1999.

The PACE Center is unique within a U.S. academic institution. It is not a pharmacy education program. Instead, it uses continuing education methods and approaches to expand the practice skills of pharmacy personnel in the development community abroad. In 2000, the center won an award for excellence in international programming in continuing education from the Learning Resources Network, a premier association in continuing education. USAID and other organizations have recognized the uniqueness of this unit and the level of excellence at which its staff seeks to perform.

The application of experience and knowledge is highlighted by the opportunity to lead HUCE's collaboration, via the PACE Center, to implement three programs under the U.S. President's Emergency Plan for AIDS Relief (PEPFAR) funding: the Global HIV/AIDS Initiative Nigeria (GHAIN) in West Africa, Regional Outreach Addressing AIDS Through Development Strategies (ROADS) in Central and East Africa, and the Twinning Project in Ethiopia. The GHAIN project, a PEPFAR flagship project, includes a focus on pharmacy services at the community level to improve pharmacists' contributions to the fight against HIV/AIDS. Under the ROADS project, pharmacy or drug shop personnel in Central and East Africa have had their knowledge base of HIV/AIDS strengthened. The Twinning Project, conducted with the American International Health Alliance, focuses on improving preservice education and strengthening curricula to enhance indigenous pharmacy education and pharmacists' contributions to the fight against HIV/AIDS. At my retirement in July 2008, it was noted that through these projects more than 1,200 pharmacy or drug shop personnel in West, Central, and East Africa have fortified their knowledge base in HIV/AIDS.

Time did not allow for many program and project reports or presentations at conferences to be in the official literature. Of note, however, are two: a presentation at the Midyear Clinical Meeting of the American Society of Health-System Pharmacists[3] and the overview focus on the use of pharmacist and other human resource needs in the fight against the HIV/AIDS pandemic.[4] Being a pharmacist with training in public health has shaped my story and given me strong leverage to apply my pharmacist's knowledge around the world.

I have loved being a pharmacist! ●

Notes

1. Galloway SP, Cain RM, Kahn JS. *Pharmacy and the Poor.* Washington, D.C.: American Pharmaceutical Association, 1971.

2. Cain RM, Khan JS. The pharmacist as a member of the health team. *Am J Public Health.* 1971;61:2223–8.

3. King R, Oqua D. Influence of a global public health program on advancing pharmacy practice in Nigeria, 2008 ASHP Midyear Clinical Meeting, Educational Session Abstracts 212–6, Orlando, Florida.

4. King RC, Fomundam HN. Remodeling pharmaceutical care in Sub-Saharan Africa (SSA) amidst human resources challenges and the HIV/AIDS pandemic. *Int J Health Plann Manage.* April 22, 2009; Epub ahead of print. 10.1002/hpm.982.

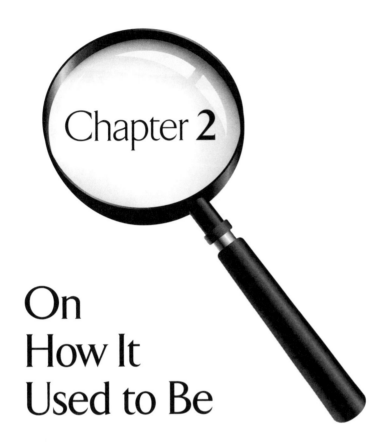

Chapter 2

On
How It
Used to Be

People are hungry for stories. It's part of our very being. Storytelling is a form of history, of immortality too. It goes from one generation to another.

—Studs Terkel

Then and Now—Mostly Then

Robert A. Lytle, RPh

Since I have been a retail pharmacist for more than 40 years, I would like to take this opportunity to tell the younger pharmacists what it was like back then. I'm sure if, as a recent graduate in 1968, I had listened to a man about to retire, he (pharmacists were almost exclusively male then) could have regaled me with "What it was like back when I started" stories that would have made my hair stand on end. No one did (or at least, I wasn't listening), but I think it would have been valuable, or at least interesting, information, as I'm hoping my recollections dispensed here are.

Rather than stating the obvious by comparing the "now" aspect with the old, you can draw your own conclusions about the differences between the two. I will simply describe the "then" part as it was in 1968. I can tell you this: Practically nothing in a modern pharmacy even closely resembles anything I learned in college.

If this sounds like another "walked uphill both ways from school" story, it's not. In some ways, retail pharmacy was much more difficult back then, but in others, it was far simpler.

In 1968, we spent most of our time—after deciphering the doctor's handwriting—typing labels on a manual typewriter. That feat completed, we affixed them to bottles by licking the yucky adhesive on the back. You don't even do that with postage stamps anymore.

I used a Bates counter to number new prescriptions and applied a date stamp to record refills, hand initialing each for good measure.

Patient profiles did not exist—pulling up charts to check for incompatibilities was impossible. Additionally, we did not type the name of the drug on the label, and we were not allowed to discuss the drug or its activity with the patient. Both were considered a breach of patient–doctor trust. If a person landed in a hospital's emergency room with a suspected overdose, the hospital staff would have to contact the drugstore and ask what a certain bottle with a certain number contained—if the store were open at the time. If not, the hospital staff had no means of determining the possible offending agent.

Naming the drug on the label was a major breakthrough, one that most doctors viewed as stepping on their professional toes. Their "Do as you're told" attitude toward their patients was a centuries-old philosophy. That attitude changed very slowly in the late 1960s, allowing patients to know what was being done to their bodies.

Back then, if a patient wanted a refill, he or she would have to call in the number or bring in the bottle. The pharmacist would then pull the original prescription, check to make sure refills were allowed, date-stamp the back to show it had been refilled, type a new label (or use the old bottle and label), and count the pills. The whole process was extremely labor intensive and provided the pharmacy a very small profit—competition with the many other local drugstores saw to that, and competition, based almost entirely on price, was fierce.

This issue brings me to a major point.

I have long believed that insurance-based prescription coverage has led to the enormous escalation of health care costs. It has long been the practice that the ultimate consumer (your customer) pays only a small portion of the actual cost of a drug—the copay. This system gave the drug companies the ability to raise their prices with impunity, and with the lid off, prices skyrocketed. Nobody noticed except the pharmacists and the sponsors—the "General Motors" of the world who actually paid the price for the inflated drug costs.

As a result, when a generically equivalent drug would come along, there was a natural resistance by customers to accept it. Why should they, when they could pay one, low copay whether the product they received was brand or generic? Over the years, public opinion, mercifully, has changed. However, pharmacists must keep both brand and generic products on the shelves to accommodate the rare request for the expensive version. When the pills go out of date, we are stuck with them. Perhaps I have delved too deeply into this thorny issue, but it is one that has bugged me my entire career. Because this is my one chance to let the world know how I feel, I'm letting fly.

To get back to the original topic, my first job out of pharmacy school brought a paltry wage of 5 dollars an hour. True, gas was about 35 cents a gallon, and a good hamburger ran about 30 cents. So, multiply everything by 10, and that's about where we are right now. Our wages are still paltry, especially when considering our responsibilities and the life-and-death decisions we make every day.

Drug salesmen back then (again, all men) were almost all pharmacists themselves and were a valued source for product information. They supplied samples of new drugs and were able to take back slow-moving products. We shared with them the camaraderie of kindred spirits. A salesperson's primary role now seems to be passing out coupons—the very bane of a retail pharmacist's existence.

As far as ownership of a drugstore, a pharmacist had to be a 51 percent stockholder. Although some chains existed, there were very few, because, to be legal, each store in a chain had to have a pharmacist as majority owner of each unit.

In retrospect, retail pharmacy wasn't all bad, but then, it wasn't all good either. As changes occurred, some of them made life simpler and some made it harder. Progress is like that—and life goes on. Hopefully, there will always be room for the independent pharmacy. ●

We Have Come a Long Way

William O. Hiner Jr., MS, RPh

In 1968, at Walson Army Hospital at Fort Dix, New Jersey, I was a young U.S. Army pharmacy officer attempting to initiate a sterile products and IV additive program. In addition to making presentations to Department of Nursing personnel to introduce this concept, I set about visiting several nursing stations to review physicians' orders for IV medications, because we did not see these orders in the pharmacy with our traditional floor stock system.

On one occasion, I was challenged by an orthopedic surgeon who wanted to know who I was and why I was on the nursing unit. I explained what I was doing, to which he replied that his father was a pharmacist who entered pharmacy during the Prohibition years for the purpose of gaining access to alcoholic beverages, which were still available for medical purposes at the time. He went on to berate me and my profession, saying that the doctors had no need for pharmacists' input on nursing units. I figured that this surely was only his personal opinion, probably reflecting his poor opinion of his father.

I continued my survey and noted an order calling for the admixture of tetracycline and hydrocortisone in the same IV bottle. Yes, we had only bottles back in the day. I advised the nurse that this would precipitate, and she subsequently relayed this information to the prescriber, who responded that she should prepare the IV as ordered. This admixture did indeed precipitate. An incident report was written, and it noted that the pharmacist cautioned against mixing these medications. During this same survey, I discovered penicillin G premixed by a nurse and stored in the unit refrigerator for several days. I expressed concern that it would decompose as a result of hydrolysis.

While I was giving my proposal for the pharmacy IV additive program, I was asked by the hospital commander if the program could be implemented without the laminar airflow hood I had requested. Fortunately, my immediate boss, who had been a cardiologist with the National Aeronautics and Space Administration (NASA), was supportive when he realized that this filter device had originated with NASA. Eventually, with enthusiastic support of nursing personnel and a few senior physicians in the chain of command, we established one of the first of three such IV additive programs in the U.S. Army Medical Department.

During the next 24 years of military pharmacy practice, I was honored to participate in the implementation and formal studies of unit-dose drug distribution, computer automation of pharmacy information systems, and clinical pharmacy services. These years were perhaps the most dynamic for the development of hospital pharmacy practice. Now, with over 40 years of active practice, I am grateful to have seen our profession become so respected in the nation's health care system. ●

Liquor Carbonis Detergens—Oh My!

Mary Shue, RPh

When I first got my pharmacist license, I was working for a university student health service. The chief pharmacist had a real love for compounding, and I was selected as the compounding pharmacist. I'll always remember the worst thing I had to compound—coal tar solution, or liquor carbonis detergens.

The whole process was messy and sticky. First, I had to measure out crude coal tar (yup, just like it sounds) and put it in a jar with washed sand. Then I added alcohol and polysorbate 80 and let it macerate for about a week on a shaker. When that process was finished, I decanted and filtered the solution. This solution was mixed with a shampoo to make—you guessed it—coal tar shampoo. It was such a mess to clean up, too. Nothing but more alcohol would do the trick.

To this day, when I smell tar on blacktop in the heat of the summer, I always think about liquor carbonis detergens. •

The First Computerized Pharmacy

Warren D. Winston, RPh

In 1967, I started my independent pharmacy, Winston's Pharmacy, A Professional Pharmacy, in my hometown of Pittsfield, Illinois, a small farming community in the Land of Lincoln. This pharmacy was one of the first American Pharmacists Association (APhA)–recognized Pharmaceutical Centers in Illinois.

I had a dream of using this new "thing" called a computer in my retail pharmacy. I knew nothing about software or hardware, and I had no computer program. So I called a friend who was a student in engineering at the University of Illinois and asked if she could write the computer program. I took along twin brothers from our high school to learn with me. There, on the Urbana campus that gave birth to the fictional computer HAL from the movie *2001: A Space Odyssey*, we dreamed up our computer system. Within a month, we were ready to start.

The local Farm Bureau, which had the only computer in the county, agreed to let me use its IBM mainframe each night. During the workday, my secretary or I would type numbers into a hand-drawn spreadsheet, including patient identification, date, prescription number, and national drug code. Each night, one of us took the spreadsheets to the Farm Bureau. There, a secretary typed all the data into a key punch reader. The punch cards were run through the bureau's computer using our pharmacy program to produce our records. The next day, we picked up printouts of inventory control, accounts payable, patient records, and drug interactions.

At the end of the first year, I sent out "patient profiles" to all of my customers, listing their total prescription costs, what prescriptions they had filled, and the dates of new and refilled prescriptions. They were astounded. They had never seen such a record—and from a computer! For those wanting a tax record, the printout was money from heaven.

I operated my pharmacy from 1967 to 1972 using this system the entire time, and I believe it was the first in the country. In fact, Dr. William Apple, past executive director of APhA and my mentor, once confirmed to me, "Yours was the first retail computerized pharmacy in the United States."

Today, with computers being ubiquitous, this idea doesn't seem particularly innovative. However, at the time, filling in those spreadsheets and driving to the Farm Bureau were part of a new and cutting-edge technology that eventually would completely change pharmacy practice. ●

A Bottle from Bethlehem

Lynn Harrelson, BPharm, FASCP

Gloria Hartman Doughty grew up in Bethlehem, Pennsylvania, and during a return visit in the 1960s, she attended an estate sale involving the contents of the Rau Drug Company, founded in 1743. Gloria noticed a beautiful little alcohol bottle with a gold label. She bought it and a few other items.

At the time of the sale, the Rau Drug Company had been the oldest continuously operating pharmacy in the United States. Sadly, the company's items were being sold off piece by piece. These historically significant pieces, which depicted the rich history of pharmacy's contributions to the citizens of Pennsylvania and the profession, would soon be scattered. Rescuing the little bottle sparked Gloria's passion for preserving pharmacy artifacts from days gone by. However, it was not the beginning of her interest in the history of pharmacy.

As a pharmacy student in the 1950s, Gloria was introduced to Dr. George Urdang from the University of Wisconsin College of Pharmacy. Dr. Urdang was the founder of the American Institute of the History of Pharmacy and a recognized author of books and articles on world pharmacy history. He signed one of his books and gave it to Gloria, opening her eyes to the rich heritage of her profession and inspiring her to begin collecting early pharmacy items.

While Gloria was employed in her first pharmacist position with Hubbard and Curry Prescription Druggists, which had opened in 1912 in Lexington, Kentucky, the owners furthered her interest in pharmacy memorabilia. They gave her several apothecary bottles, and her collection grew even more one special Christmas when they gave her a three-tiered, handblown apothecary show globe from Blenko Glass Company in West Virginia. Later, when Hubbard and Curry was remodeled in the 1960s, the owners gave her two glass, marble-based showcases, into which she gladly placed her growing apothecary collection.

Gloria's apothecary collection complemented the collection of medicinal plant specimens assembled by her husband, Dick Doughty, a pharmacognosist. As fate would have it, many times their passion for collecting crossed paths.

Originally published in the *Kentucky Pharmacist*, January 2009. Adapted with permission from Kentucky Pharmacists Association.

During their first trip to Europe, her husband met with Burroughs Wellcome concerning his plant research, and Gloria visited with the Wellcome Museum's curator of ancient glass. While touring a vast collection of glass from Egyptian tombs dating back to 2000 BC, Gloria started thinking about preserving pharmacy memorabilia for future generations.

Gloria was appointed to the Kentucky Board of Pharmacy in 1969, and later, she was commissioned to write the history of the organization. She spent several years collecting material from the board's archives in Frankfort. During one of her trips to Frankfort, she learned of a recently closed pharmacy in Wilmore with great fixtures. The owners of the building were looking for a new use for the site, possibly a pharmacy museum. This news prompted Gloria and a friend with business experience to incorporate the Kentucky Renaissance Pharmacy Museum and Fountain as a nonprofit museum. Her dream of establishing a pharmacy museum in Kentucky was beginning to be realized, although the Wilmore pharmacy didn't fit the bill.

The recently closed site was attractive, but because it was in the small city of Wilmore, it would not get much foot traffic. Gloria and others on the museum's board discovered that the Old Fayette County Courthouse in Lexington, the second-largest city in the state, was being transformed into a complex of history museums and exhibits. Gloria and the others petitioned the Lexington Metro Government for space in the complex, and after meeting with every pertinent committee and the mayor, they were successful in securing a suite of five rooms on the ground floor.

With the support and sponsorship of the Blue Grass Pharmacists Association, Jefferson County Academy of Pharmacy, Kentucky Pharmacists Association, University of Kentucky College of Pharmacy, other pharmacy groups, and many dedicated, hardworking individuals, the Kentucky Renaissance Pharmacy Museum opened in June 2005. Attendees at the joint meeting of the Kentucky Pharmacists Association and the Kentucky Society of Health-System Pharmacists visited the museum during its ribbon cutting and opening weekend.

The museum has a special tie with a Lexington pharmacy. In the 1970s, Gloria discovered that the Bradley Drug Store on Main Street was being torn down. Remembering the Rau Drug Company, Gloria called her friend and former Lexington mayor Foster Pettit, who owned the building. She asked him for the glass panels on the cupola, and with the help of several students from the University of Kentucky College of Pharmacy, two panels were rescued. These panels dated back to 1889, when pharmacist Albert Johns built the building. One panel, red and white with a mortar-and-pestle design, now hangs in the Kentucky Renaissance Pharmacy Museum and was the inspiration for the museum's logo.

Just as Gloria had dreamed, the museum displays major collections of memorabilia representing Kentucky pharmacy from the late 1700s, 1800s, and 1900s. Many of her days are spent securing and organizing the various collections that have been donated to the museum for preservation. Most weekends she can be found at the museum greeting members of the public and sharing with them the history of pharmacy in Kentucky. Consistent with the museum's mission and Gloria's passion, the museum has enlightened visitors from more than 40 states and every continent.

Thanks to Gloria and that little bottle from Bethlehem, myriad historical items can be seen on display at the Kentucky Renaissance Pharmacy Museum. ●

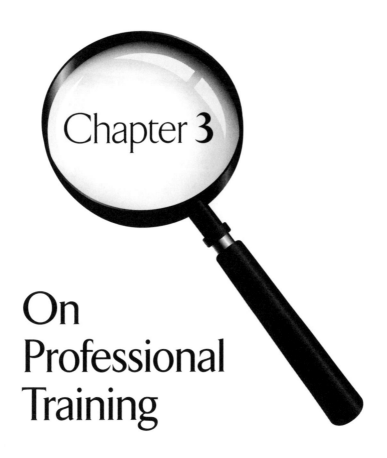

Chapter 3

On Professional Training

*Life is my college. May I graduate well,
and earn some honors!*

—Louisa May Alcott

Pharmacy School at 40-Something

Mary Ann Mobilian, PharmD candidate

I lay on the sofa in my parents' living room, not wanting to open my eyes. It had been a rough night. My sisters and I were taking care of my mother with the help of hospice; I still couldn't believe that she was dying from brain cancer. Even though she was in a semicoma, her pain from the tumor's growth required morphine regularly. Last night had been my night to check on my mother every couple of hours and give her pain medication as needed. It had been a restless night for her, and I was exhausted when the alarm went off.

Still fighting opening my eyes to the world, I was thinking about all the things I needed to do that day, when a vivid image of angels hovering over my mother came into my thoughts. I tried to read their expressions and wondered if they would still be there if I opened my eyes; they were not. The serenity of the image was soon forgotten as I went to work gathering the medications and new bedding for my mother. Later that morning, I noticed my mother was very restless, so I took her hand; it was at that moment, she breathed her last breath. Our family was consumed by our loss, and it wasn't until later in the day that I suddenly recalled the image of the angels. We all found great comfort in the angels being there to help our mother make her final journey.

The loss of my mother forced me to consider my own mortality and what I would leave behind. At the time, I was regional vice president for a REIT, or real estate investment trust, and it was financially, but not personally, rewarding. I realized I wanted more of a "legacy" than working 60 to 80 hours per week and making a lot of money for a big corporation. Thinking about more rewarding career options, I remembered how some of the people who took care of my mother were the highlight of her day. They always remembered her name, smiled warmly, and showed her respect in the midst of invasive procedures. They also helped family members deal with a terminal diagnosis, the demands of being caregivers, and the unbearable emotion of seeing the ravages of cancer steal away the life of someone you love dearly. But could I really make such a dramatic career change at 43 years old?

Originally published in the *Journal of the American Pharmacists Association*, 2009;49:47–2. Adapted with permission.

Going back to college as a nontraditional student would be stressful enough, but going for a doctorate in pharmacy, I must be insane! My original goal was to become a radiation technician, but that program dissolved after losing the instructor. A counselor encouraged me to apply to the new University of Florida College of Pharmacy's satellite program right here in Jacksonville, Florida. I was hesitant at first, because I really wanted more patient contact. But after talking with the counselor, I realized that there were a lot of opportunities to make a difference in someone's life by being involved in his or her health care as a pharmacist. Perhaps if I had known how competitive getting into the program was, I would have been too intimidated to even try.

Finishing all the prerequisite courses was challenging; organic chemistry was almost my undoing. After my first organic chemistry exam, I found myself in the professor's office, tearfully asking how I could improve my grade. She smiled at me, explained the concept of curving grades (turns out the class average was in the mid-50s), and told me that my grade was in the top of the class!

Finally, the day came to apply and *wait*. I was convinced that the admissions office would take one look at my application and wonder what kind of a midlife crisis would drive someone to apply to the college at 45 years old, thinking, "Doesn't she realize that she will be 50 when she graduates?" At times, I wondered the same thing. When I did get my acceptance letter, it was one of the proudest moments of my life.

The first year began with orientation. The "type A" personalities that filled the auditorium were forewarned that their grades may take a turn for the worse, but resuscitation was always possible. I recall thinking that I didn't need to listen when they were explaining how many D's we were allowed before getting booted from the program, because the worst grade I had made was a C (in, you guessed it, organic chemistry). I was in for a rude awakening, and year one was just the beginning.

The second year was by far the most difficult. My husband, John, had to undergo seven back surgeries, five at Mayo Clinic in Jacksonville. I spent most of my days reading and studying for exams in hospital rooms, in fact, so much so, that the physicians started giving me pop quizzes on whatever subject I was studying. Even with massive doses of coffee (why don't they make an IV dosage form?), my 40-something brain, with neurons firing at maximum capacity, struggled to keep up. If it wasn't for the love and support of my family, friends, and fellow students, I wonder if I would have made it through that year. On those occasions when I felt like giving up, a little voice reminded me of what I had always preached to my sons: "Winners never quit; quitters never win." (Don't you hate it when your own words come back to haunt you?)

Year three brought different challenges because it was geared toward preparing students for our upcoming rotations. Pharmacotherapy classes had students participate in mock consultations, answering questions and making therapeutic recommendations—all while being recorded. If you've never had the experience of viewing a recording of yourself trying to appear intelligent while sweating bullets, be sure to add this to your list of "Not now, not evers." This humiliating process taught us two important lessons: how to say "I don't know, but I'll get back to you" when we didn't know the answer and that most of the time, we didn't know the answer.

I'm now in the final year and going through rotations. I can see the light at the end of the tunnel (but only with my reading glasses). Rotations are going great, and I've learned a lot from all my preceptors. In fact, the reason I'm writing this article is that my current preceptor at Mayo Clinic (how ironic that I'm here as a rotation student) offers students the option of writing an article for publication. I have to admit that at first, writing an article was intimidating, but rotations are all about meeting new challenges and learning from them.

Writing this article made me think about what my experience in pharmacy school has taught me. I learned just how remarkably supportive and loving my husband is. I've learned some people don't believe in challenging themselves after a certain age, but your friends will admire you for the very things others think are senseless. I've learned that I don't have to worry about what's going to happen when the next generation takes over. Even though most of my classmates are young enough to be my children, they are dedicated to academic and professional excellence.

I've also thought about what my patients have taught me. I've learned from them how rewarding pharmacy practice can be. One patient at a drugstore chain brought me a starfish from the beach for helping with her depression medications. Another patient at a local medical center requested I come back and counsel his wife on warfarin because he was so impressed with how I explained everything in layman's terms.

The lessons taught to me by pharmacists are what I hope to emulate in my own practice once I graduate. I learned that the principle of giving back is alive and well in preceptors, professors, and fellow practitioners and that most pharmacists chose the profession out of a desire to help others. I've learned that this profession is one of the few in which perfection isn't a goal but a standard of practice.

I began this pursuit out of a desire to make a difference before I take my final journey with the angels. Now, however, after writing this article, I realize that I've had angels with me all along. ●

A Story of Getting Accepted to Pharmacy School

John Backus, PharmD

I was in my second year of undergraduate studies (in biology) when I decided to send out applications to pharmacy school en masse. The previous year, I had applied to only one pharmacy school (naively thinking that my good grades and good essay-writing ability would get me in) and had been rejected. At the time, I was dating a girl whose mother was a career counselor, and she gave me several brochures from pharmacy schools across the United States and Canada. (The thought did cross my mind that maybe she was so helpful because she wanted me to move away from her daughter.)

For 2 straight months, every single day, I filled out application forms, got reference letters, wrote essays, crossed all the t's, and dotted all the i's. On top of this, I had my regular undergraduate course studies, which was a full-time job in and of itself. Finally, at the end of the 2 months, with 2 weeks to spare before most application deadlines, I had completed and mailed applications to every pharmacy school in the United States east of Nebraska and every pharmacy school in Canada. It was an expensive and tiring proposition.

On the Sunday afternoon after I had sent out all my applications, I was sitting on my couch watching football and trying to relax. I looked to my side and saw one last brochure with application materials in it that I had forgotten to fill out. The thought of doing one more essay or begging for one more letter of reference was unbearable. So, I told myself, "I'll fill out this application, but if it asks for an essay or a reference letter, it's going in the trash." As I watched the game, I filled out the application. After 15 minutes, it was done, and no essays or reference letters were required, although it did ask for an official copy of my transcripts. I mailed it the next morning.

As the months went by, I got rejection letter upon rejection letter. All of that hard work, all of those nights spent in the library writing application essays, all of those reference letters I had to collect—everything seemed to be a waste. What was I going to do with my life? I didn't want to become a biologist. I would have to grow a shaggy beard, wear sloppy clothes, eat granola, drive a hippie van, and spend my summers in mosquito-infested forests. My grades were decent. Why didn't any pharmacy school want me? If I can't get in, who does?

Then, it happened. I finally got an acceptance letter. From where, you ask? None other than the school whose application I had filled out in 15 minutes while watching the Buffalo Bills get trounced. It had been the very last application I had filled out, and I didn't think it had been my best hope for acceptance. I assumed my qualifications fit several other schools better, but all of them rejected me.

My first thought was, "Is this place legit?" After looking into it, I found out that it was the oldest pharmacy school in the United States and very highly rated. As it turned out, the year I applied, it was expanding its pharmacy program and accepting more undergraduates and transfers to fill the new spaces. I didn't need a bachelor's degree to get in; good grades in my 2 years of undergraduate studies up to that point reflected my abilities adequately. It also didn't hurt that I had extracurricular activities on my resume to "round me out" as a person.

Four years later, I graduated with a doctor of pharmacy degree and a 3.6 grade point average. I moved to Florida and have lived the "Florida lifestyle" ever since. It just goes to show that you never know when luck (or divine intervention) will trump everything else and take your life on a path you never could have imagined. I met many wonderful friends during my years in pharmacy school and had the opportunity to visit and work in numerous interesting places—a summer interning on Martha's Vineyard was a highlight. None of it would have happened if I had given up after receiving so many rejection letters. The old saying really is true: If at first you don't succeed, try, try again. ●

The Crosswalk

Peter A. Chyka, PharmD

For three decades I've watched a scene as regular as a heartbeat,
Where young student pharmacists have crossed a busy, urban street.
Briskly, they crossed this path to reach their challenging classes,
Eyes bright, backpacks full, feet fearlessly marching with the masses.
Some silent, others not as they discuss what they've been taught,
Either way, to reach their career goal they must take the crosswalk.

Fresh-faced students in their first year of school,
Carefree, excited, confident—not wanting to look the fool.
Boldly, they cross that street alone or as an overwhelming herd,
No attention paid to the signal, traffic, people, nor the rest of the world.
Concentration fixed on the task of the day and the degree they've sought,
It makes little difference in their step if they must make the crosswalk.

By end of the first semester when it's time for a well-deserved break,
Their steps are more measured and watchful so as not to make a mistake.
They have seen and felt the unexpected for which they were unprepared.
Sick people, drug errors, ethical concerns, all part of a profession now shared.
The street still looks exciting, but feels more humbling and danger-fraught.
Compassion and consideration for others are now part of their daily crosswalk. ●

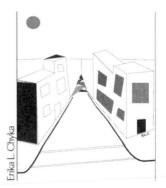

Erika L. Chyka

What My Pharmacy Mentor Couldn't Teach Me, but Did

Jessica Stovel, Hon BSc, BScPhm

As I entered my final year of pharmacy school, I faced a familiar quandary: In what direction should I go? Before deciding on pharmacy as a prospective career, I spent 5 years at university completing an undergraduate degree in the sciences. I had a love for chemistry, research, and linguistics and social communications and specialized in all three areas. I delved earnestly into each discipline in the hopes of finding my niche. However, as my understanding of each grew, so too did my interest. Increasingly, I was reluctant to commit to just one.

A doctoral student in the research lab where I worked had the insight to encourage me to apply to pharmacy school, because being a pharmacist would enable me to combine all three loves—a perfect match. I eagerly went through the pharmacy program, but as I progressed, I realized that I had many potential avenues to explore: community pharmacy, where I would have the reward of building lasting relationships; hospital pharmacy, where I could focus on immediate care; or industry or government, where I might pursue my love for research. Which offered the most rewarding career path? After much reflection, and not without some trepidation, I decided to complete a year of residency upon graduation. Hospital pharmacy seemed to coincide most closely with my interests, with the added benefit of leaving my options open.

The journey began one evening as I was preparing for a 13-month stay in a new city that I knew was going to be a life-altering experience: my hospital residency program in London, Ontario. As I was packing, I received an e-mail from a pharmacist, JL, at my placement hospital welcoming me and wishing me the best as I set forth on my new career. I was touched by his thoughtfulness and kindness in making me feel welcome before I had even arrived. Little did I imagine that this extended hand would be the first of so many proffered by JL, who would become my mentor as I embarked on my new career.

I was fortunate to meet JL on the second day of my residency. His enthusiasm, charisma, and love of teaching immediately captured my attention. He made such a strong impression that I quickly rearranged my schedule so that I could complete as much time as possible in psychiatry, his clinical area. As it happened, psychiatry was my first clinical rotation. It was a unique experience resulting from a combination of JL's dedicated teaching and his desire to expose his residents to as many opportunities as possible.

As my teacher, he helped me develop and refine my therapeutic thought process by consistently walking me through his thought process when discussing patient cases and then seeking my contribution. He also sought every opportunity to enrich my residency experience, although he was under no obligation to do so. The first event was a chance to participate in a national teleconference sponsored by a pharmaceutical company to discuss its launch of a new psychiatric medication. Over the next 11 months, I had many opportunities to attend continuing education events and conferences, participate in medical classes taught by pharmacists at the university, give presentations to family and patient groups, and attend professional development events for leading practitioners in the health care community.

In the course of all these activities, JL was diligent in introducing me to his contacts so that I too could start to build a professional network. These unexpected opportunities significantly broadened my knowledge, reinforced what I learned from my clinical rotations, and built my confidence.

In addition, JL took the time during my clinical rotation with him to discuss his career and the various twists and turns it had taken to lead him to his current position. These conversations were invaluable in assessing my professional opportunities. He helped me plan my career path after residency and counseled me on my decision to accept a position as a pediatric pharmacist. As I ventured into this complex and specialized field, he was always there to support me by listening and discussing concerns and obstacles that arose. His insights and sound advice enabled me to cope with the many challenges on this service with growing assurance in my judgment and decisions.

JL also challenged me to think about my long-term career path. He listened to my hopes and aspirations and used this understanding to find unique opportunities for me that would give me a taste of my dreams. I first realized his belief in me when he told me that a research assignment he had given me was actually a question to be answered in a column in a professional medical resource. He invited me to take what I had written, combine it with his thoughts, and publish it with him. I was flattered that he had trust in my abilities.

Over the past 2 years, he has given me other extraordinary opportunities to write with him, collaborate on research projects, develop a continuing education Web module, and present publicly together. Beyond helping me fine-tune critical skills, these tasks greatly improved my poise and professional assurance. Through JL's mentoring, I realize that it is indeed possible to combine my passions (research, teaching, and writing) with hospital practice. As a result of all that he has taught me, I am confident that I have chosen the right road and look forward to the multitude of possibilities that lie before me as a hospital pharmacist.

In addition to professional mentorship, JL has dedicated much time to guiding my personal development. He has imparted much wisdom, teaching me to be self-aware, to be giving and thankful, to embrace change, to strive for excellence, and to think positively. In this last regard, one of the most valuable skills that I have learned is to search for the positives from an otherwise seemingly negative situation. This perspective helped me immensely throughout residency and continues to assist me to deal with difficult situations that arise in my new clinical practice.

I will be forever grateful for the knowledge, skills, opportunities, and support that JL has given me over the past 2 years, as well as for his faith in me. However, I believe that the most important value that I derived from our mentoring relationship lies in what he could not teach me. I have learned far more than he could ever consciously impart from having an opportunity to work closely with him and observe him. In his daily practice and personal interactions, I have seen the combination of attributes that make JL a unique practitioner and special person. He is caring and dedicated. He consistently goes above and beyond what is required to ensure patients receive the best patient care possible. He routinely reaches out beyond his service to assist patients in need, as well as those who have sought him out for help. He is visionary. He is always thinking ahead of the curve and outside of the box. As just one example, he not only holds patient medication groups in his practice, but he facilitates these sessions in such a manner that the patients teach each other as much as he teaches them.

JL is determined. He is willing to take any risk, no matter what the potential fallout, to advance his practice or achieve a goal in which he believes. He is generous. He provides deserving students and residents with opportunities to develop themselves and prove their abilities. He treats everyone with respect. Regardless of status or social position, he relates to everyone as an equal and does not judge. JL has initiative. He strives to improve himself through continuing education, research, and writing. Of particular note, he has charisma. His engaging personality and wit enable him to easily build rapport and patient relationships, win the trust of his patients, and captivate his audience when he presents or teaches.

Albert Einstein said, "Setting an example is not the main means of influencing another; it is the only means." As I move forward in the profession, I realize that in whatever direction my career ultimately takes, my success will depend more on what I have learned observing my mentor than on what he taught me. It is JL's particular combination of qualities and attributes that shapes his professionalism, and I admire him for the pharmacist and person he is. He represents the pharmacist that I aspire to be. ●

Hooked on Teaching: My Journey to Academic Pharmacy

Ashley W. Ellis, PharmD

When I entered pharmacy school at the University of Mississippi in 2003, I was surrounded by students committed to pharmacy, striving for the best grades. They were students used to receiving the best grades at the institutions from which they came. We spent all 3 years of classroom learning side by side. We studied at the school until the wee hours of the morning and celebrated after weeks of daily exams ended. I enjoyed learning and I knew pharmacy was the field I needed to be in, but I could not shake the feeling that everybody else understood all of our complex coursework better than I did. It seemed like I had to study harder and longer hours than those around me, and I didn't always get straight A's, even with the extra work.

As I entered rotations in my final year of pharmacy school, I was surprised how easily the knowledge came back to me when preceptors asked me questions. Being in different clinical settings helped me put the pieces together and reinforced what I learned during all of those late-night study sessions. Halfway through the year, my confidence in each rotation had grown. In January, I had a pharmacy administration practice experience back on the campus of the university. This rotation focused on teaching, learning styles, and pedagogy. I'm not sure exactly why I picked this rotation in my third year, but it seemed interesting.

At the beginning of the rotation, my preceptor excitedly explained the topics of discussion, readings, and projects that were due over the course of our 6 weeks together. We discussed how she came to academia and discovered we both had parents who were educators who had an influence over our career choices. As I discovered more about why my teachers had taught in the way that they did, how test questions were written, how objectives for lectures were carefully selected, and how learning styles influenced the adult learner, I had a newfound respect for the educators in my professional training. On the last day of the rotation as we went over my evaluation, my preceptor told me that she thought I should become a teacher. My first thought was, "Are you crazy? I'm not even the best student in my class. What could anybody learn from me?" I took her words away with me as I finished rotations and entered into my community pharmacy practice residency.

In my residency, I was able to teach several lecture hours and completed a teaching certificate program. Being around pharmacy students and academia brought up my past preceptor's suggestion again, and as I prepared for job interviews, I realized she was right all along. My first job after residency was as an assistant professor of pharmacy practice at Shenandoah University. I taught lectures in the therapeutics classes and coordinated a lab for first-year pharmacy students in communications and patient counseling. Being new to teaching, I used the active-learning techniques I learned on my rotation and in the teaching certificate program. Some ideas worked and some didn't, but I found I was enjoying my job more than I could have imagined. The idea that I could help shape future pharmacists to go out and advance the profession invigorated me to try to package information for students in the best way possible.

If that wasn't exciting enough, I discovered that my alma mater had a new position open and was interested in having a community pharmacy faculty member apply for it. I applied and was offered the job. I'm just getting started in my field, and the opportunities seem endless. I am developing a new course that focuses on skills needed by pharmacy students to practice in a real-world pharmacy environment and provide medication therapy management services to patients with asthma and diabetes in the Mississippi Delta.

As a student on rotations, I thought the best preceptors were the ones who loved their jobs. As a pharmacist working in academic pharmacy, I can say that I am among those who love their jobs. I even have an office across the hall from one of those preceptors who not only loves her job but also has helped to shape my entire career with her encouraging words. I remember her confidence in me before I had confidence in myself and can see the evidence of what a difference it made. Her example leads me to strive to do the same for my students so that future pharmacists can go on to achieve a career that they love and to lead our profession to advance beyond our wildest dreams. ●

The Transformation of Pharmacy Students

Compiled by Sharon Connor, PharmD, and Mary Herbert, MS, MPH

The University of Pittsburgh second-year pharmacy students are required to complete a one-time service experience at a clinic for a population that is homeless or uninsured. Fear and hesitancy about their abilities and the community populations they are about to serve inevitably give way to feelings of understanding and respect for the patients, as well as a newfound confidence in themselves as emerging providers and volunteers. Their personal and professional transformations are profound and life-changing. The following comments were written by the students about their experiences.

I Had Absolutely No Idea What to Expect

"When I first pulled up to the free clinic, I was almost certain I had made a mistake. I was expecting to see a small storefront with a colorful, protective awning where I would enter into a small waiting room with a few patients sitting and relaxing. However, what I saw came as a bit of a shock. After a dimly lit walk through an alley, I found myself staring at a distant black door. When I got closer, I noticed the paper sign taped to the door that said 'Birmingham Clinic.' I walked in hesitantly, still unsure of what to expect. I squeezed through a tiny waiting area overflowing with patients.

"The quick-paced atmosphere gave me a burst of adrenaline. I bustled around with other volunteers to interview patients and check blood pressures and blood glucose readings. The environment not only thrust me into new and wonderful practices, but it also made me feel like part of a more important movement. Even though the patients came early and waited for hours to be served, I could feel their gratitude."

Everyone Deserves Dignity and Respect

"I was surprised by the willingness and interest of the patients to learn about their medications and disease states, even though most of them had other priorities, such as putting a roof over their head and finding food for their stomach. As I counseled them, I realized how much I was learning from them. I learned about their hardships and their lifestyle. I was amazed by their optimism under these circumstances. Initially, I was fearful of the homeless, but now I have learned that the homeless are not that different from us. They share the same dreams and hopes that we all do."

"One occurrence stands out in my mind. A patient brought in her two new beautiful outfits that she bought at a yard sale. She was so happy, and gleefully she said, 'Can you believe it? I only paid five dollars for each of these suits!' She was just like any other woman who enjoys shopping for good bargains."

"I came to the clinic expecting to see a desperate population. What I found, however, was a group of individuals with great pride who want to better themselves, beginning with their health."

Community Need: Through the Eyes of Pharmacy Students
"The most important lesson I learned was the lesson of need. Everyone was there to help. There was no insurance or money, no hurries or schedules, no egos involved, and everyone was treated with respect. I knew that such a need existed, but being there really drove it home for me and made me realize I take receiving health care for granted."

"The Birmingham Clinic was definitely an eye-opening experience for me. I never realized what a privilege it is to have health insurance. Having one man tell me he never goes to the doctor and has not seen one in over 30 years because he cannot afford it was a conversation that I will never forget."

"This clinic experience left me very humbled. I came to realize that there are so many things that I take for granted far too often, like my health, education, and the safety I feel."

I Am Inspired
"There was something appealing to me about health care that isn't based on profit. This experience inspired me. It allowed me to see the side of health care that I want to be a part of. I really can't wait to go back. I loved my experience."

"I absolutely cannot wait until I get another chance to volunteer in another underserved clinic!"

"When I left the clinic, I knew I wanted to spend more time volunteering there."

"As health care professionals, we all have a calling to help the underserved. To have a good society, we need to take time out of our busy schedules to reach out to those less fortunate than ourselves."

"My experience at the Birmingham Clinic has reinforced the notion that, as a health care provider, it is my role to actively participate in community health initiatives."

I Am Proud

"This is by far the most rewarding experience that I have ever had. I left feeling as though I had actually made a difference in every patient I had worked with that evening. Everyone deserves to have quality health care in our country."

"After I left the clinic, I felt a sense of pride and fulfillment because it felt really great to help people who are less fortunate and I was able to use my learned pharmacy skills to help them obtain medical care."

"I am so grateful to be able to have had this opportunity; this is a way that I could really give back and start to find ways to use the skills I am learning in a place where they are needed."

"This experience made me feel proud to be a part of the health care profession."

"When I was finished for the evening at the clinic, I had a great sense of satisfaction and pride. No matter what background people come from, what problems they have had in the past, or what their current job status might be, they are all human and all deserve our respect. A recent college graduate is not more deserving of treatment than a recovering substance abuser."

"Honestly, the experience made me feel great inside. Working with the patients was a wonderful experience. People of all shapes, sizes, and colors deserve sound medical treatment. I learned that helping people is what matters." ●

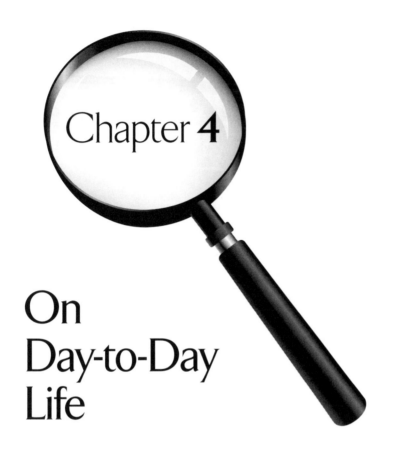

Chapter 4

On Day-to-Day Life

A piller of the community.

—**Anonymous**

Divine Dispensing

Janet Bradshaw, BSP

During one of the stages of my career, I was doing relief work for several pharmacies in the rural area that I lived in. On one particular Saturday, I had anticipated a slower day. I brought along some work that I needed to do to prepare for my Sunday school class the following day.

As I was filling a prescription for a gentleman, he asked, "Expecting a hard day?"

"No, not really," I replied, "but why do you ask?"

He pointed to my pile of books that I had stacked beside the computer and said, "I see you brought your Bible along." ●

So, You Are a Pharmacist!

Olafur Olafsson, MSc Pharm

I am not a handsome guy. Actually, I am not good looking at all. I would never have been asked to model for any fashion designer, and I would never have had a career in the film industry. So I chose a different profession: I became a pharmacist.

One day an elderly man walked into the pharmacy and asked to speak to a pharmacist. When I approached him, I realized that we had been neighbors some years earlier. He looked at me and exclaimed, "So, you are a pharmacist!"

"Yes I am," I answered rather proudly.

"Really," he said. "I always thought that you only looked like one!"

Ever since that day, I have known what a pharmacist should look like. I am reminded every time I see my pitiful reflection in the mirror. ●

Dispensed with Rocky Mountain Spring Water

Stephen L. Murley, RPh

M y first pharmacy job found me working as a decentralized pharmacist in a large urban hospital. Like many hospitals, the copy of the physician's orders provided to the pharmacy was the last page of a three-page carbonless form. In this hospital, each nurse's station had a small "pharmacy basket" where the orders were placed for the pharmacist. Because I was a newly licensed RPh, one of my nursing units enjoyed playing small pranks by placing an order for something totally bogus. I remember picking up an order for "Fleet's eye drops" once.

This particular day, I reached in the basket and pulled out an order clearly written as, "One can of beer daily with the evening meal." I looked at the nurse who had written the verbal order and said something like, "Cute."

She turned the chart on which she was writing toward me, much in the way someone would when reading to a child. She pointed at an original order with her pen and said, "This one is real." I sat down in the chair next to her and asked to see the chart.

There it was, right after the patient's admission orders. I flipped to the physician's note section to read the admission note. The patient was there for some minor cardiac procedure. (Today as I write this, I don't remember the specifics.) It was also noted that the patient had a history of alcoholism. In the plan section of the note, the doc had written, "Prevent DT." Now I understood. The goal of the daily beer was to prevent delirium tremens.

On my way back to the pharmacy, I passed the physician in the hall. I asked him about the therapy ordered. He advised that he had prevented alcohol withdrawal this way before. While lorazepam or something similar would probably do the trick, beer had some advantages: It was cheaper, and it fulfilled the patient's craving (both physically and psychologically). At the moment, treating his cardiac issue was more important than treating his alcoholism. For the patient's overall well-being, the cardiac problem had to be fixed first. Dealing with withdrawal in an unstable cardiac patient posed greater risk than maintaining the alcoholism and treating his heart.

Somewhere in this conversation, I realized the importance of working with a patient in a give-and-take method to reach treatment goals. A patient doesn't have to have everything "fixed" at once. Work with the patient, and help find that balance. The doc told me that he and the patient had discussed the options, and this course of action is what they had decided on.

Back in the pharmacy, the fridge was full of insulin, pancuronium, and other drugs, but no beer. I walked up to our materials management person and with a smile said, "I need a beer." He replied, "Me too. I can't wait until 11 pm." I then proceeded to tell him about the situation with the patient on the telemetry floor. To my surprise, he wasn't surprised. "We've dispensed beer before," he said. "Go ask the patient what kind he would like."

I knocked lightly on the patient's door and went in. I introduced myself as the pharmacist and explained that I would be the one responsible for bringing his evening beer. He was probably in his mid-70s and had crew-cut hair and rectangular wire-rimmed glasses. His nose was slightly enlarged and reddened, coordinating nicely with his red bathrobe. He joked about "brand name" versus "generic." Coors would be preferred to the white can with the word "Beer" on it. I relayed the brand request to the materials manager.

A few hours later, there was a 12-pack in our drug fridge. Hospital policy dictated that it must be labeled, so I hand-typed a label. I opted for the "Keep refrigerated" auxiliary label over the "Keep refrigerated and shake well prior to administration."

As the elevator doors opened on the telemetry floor, there was the patient, waiting, well, patiently. He took the can and padded back to his room, house shoes making the characteristic woosh-woosh sound across the floor.

And so it went for the next 4 or 5 days. As I made my 5 pm rounds, the patient would meet me at the elevator for his dose of brew. His procedure was a success, and he was discharged. The leftover cans of beer remained in the fridge. ●

While Waiting for a Third-Party Rep to Come to the Phone

Martin Niedelman, BPharm

There are days when I don't have time to go to the bathroom or eat lunch. But I can guess that cumulatively I might spend an hour or two on the phone with the third-party plans, trying to resolve a predicament. It seems a shame to waste this time. So, what can you do when you're on hold?

You could try singing, "One hundred bottles of beer on the wall, 100 bottles of beer. When one of those bottles happens to fall, there are 99 bottles of beer on the wall." You can sing this until there are no bottles of beer left. During the average call, you can usually eliminate 10–15 bottles, after pushing several buttons on the phone to get to the hold position. When you get tired of this song, you can choose several other things to do. You could recite the Gettysburg Address, play a game of solitaire, or listen to an extra inning of a baseball game. Of course, I'm exaggerating by bringing up these ideas. But you get my point. You could be filling prescriptions, counseling patients, and making extra sales out front.

You may have a phone system with two or three lines. While you are on hold, waiting for a plan representative to answer, you are tying up one line. On the second line, someone may be talking to a boyfriend or girlfriend. On the third line, a doctor may be phoning in a prescription. Anyone else calling now can't reach you.

This brings up another predicament. You have a doctor on one line, and you know the doctor is not going to wait there more than 10 seconds. If you put the third party on hold and that person answers the phone, he or she will hang up if you're not there, and you will have to go through the whole process again. If you don't talk to the doctor, the doctor may hang up and you may lose one or several prescriptions. So, what do you do? I guess you can clone yourself, so that you can speak to two people at one time. If you have one or two customers out front who need your expertise, you may have to clone yourself three or four times.

Several items could make your life easier. You should have a functioning speaker phone or a headset, so that you can do other things in the proximity of your phone. It would be wonderful if there were a universal third-party insurance card. This card could clearly state the bin number, group number, patient ID number, and the person code. Fancy ID numbers with letters mixed in with the person code should be eliminated.

Guessing whether it's a zero or the letter O is insane. I can't tell you how many times I have had to call because the group number on the card was wrong. Then the plan representative gives me a completely different one. I'm about to voice my opinion, but I refrain from doing so. I know that the person on the other end of the phone has nothing to do with the policy making of the plan, and if I yell too loudly, it may trigger an audit. So when he or she says to me, "Is there anything else I can do for you today?" I say, "No, thank you very much for your time, and enjoy your day." ●

Unexpected Help

Joanna Maudlin Pangilinan, PharmD, BCOP

It was busy in the satellite on that Wednesday night. I was the only pharmacist servicing three high-acuity medicine floors in an urban, academic hospital. Things were under control when the code was called.

"Come on, let's go!" I urged my third-year pharmacy student, who also happened to be one of my technicians that night. She wanted to see what the pharmacist did during a code.

We raced through the hallways and down the stairs, joining many others on their own pursuit to the code. We knew we had arrived when we saw a room overflowing with nurses, respiratory therapists, and physicians from many different teams.

Upon entry into the room, I saw that the patient was awake. He was having a heart attack. The physicians were trying to gather information because he had just been admitted from the emergency department.

"Are you having chest pain?" "Where does it hurt? Does it radiate anywhere?" "Are you having problems breathing?" "Can you chew this aspirin?"

The patient lay there speechlessly. All alone.

A nurse cried, "He can't understand you!"

A physician glanced up from the chart and looked around helplessly. "Does anyone speak Ukrainian?" he shouted.

The room fell silent. People looked at each other.

Beside me came a movement and then a voice. My student stepped forward and said, "I do." ●

Employee of the Month

Mike Johnson, RPh

After several years of service working as a pharmacist in my hometown community hospital, I was selected as Employee of the Month. One of the perks associated with this honor is a dedicated parking spot as close as possible to the main hospital entrance. One day when I came in for a day shift (7:00 am to 3:30 pm), I was disturbed to find that someone had parked in my space. Not knowing who had done this or how to fix the problem, I decided to park as close as possible to the rear of the offending vehicle, making it impossible for the person to leave without my assistance.

I proceeded into the building and began my usual shift duties, one of which was communicating with the night-shift pharmacist before he departed. I related my actions to him, and we both had a chuckle about the whole situation, and he left for home to catch up on his sleep. A few minutes later I received a call from this same night-shift pharmacist saying a nurse was "trapped" in my Employee of the Month parking space and she would like for me to let her out so she could go home. I told him I would be right down.

I asked the guilty nurse why she chose my spot to park in; there were many empty parking spaces only a few feet away. She proceeded to give me a very sad story of how she had been called into the critical care unit for a code in the middle of the night and was never able to leave or get back to move her vehicle before I got to work.

I looked around and noticed the number of empty spaces all over the parking lot, some of which were the clergy-only spaces right next to the one reserved for the Employee of the Month. I told her I would be glad to let her go home this time, but if she parked in the space again (at least while I was Employee of the Month), she might be better off taking a chance on a clergy spot. ●

Amitriptyline in the Coffee

Michael J. Schuh, PharmD, MBA

While working in a busy chain pharmacy some years ago, I noticed something hard in my mouth after lunch. Thinking it was something left over from lunch—perhaps a bone—I spit it out. Behold! It was a 25-mg amitriptyline tablet! Because I didn't take amitriptyline, I retraced the events of my day (now called a root cause analysis). That morning, I had counted a large number of amitriptyline tablets in the Kirby Lester pill counter and had my spill-proof coffee mug near the machine. While dumping tablets, I didn't notice one had bounced out of the machine onto the top of my cup, ready to lodge between a space in my teeth on the next sip of coffee. How the tablet survived not being dissolved, swallowed during the rest of the cup of coffee, or eaten during lunch I'll never know. ●

What We Really Do

Robert A. Lytle, RPh

When I first noticed the call for pharmacists' stories, I thought, "I can do this." I've been a pharmacist for 40 years and owned my own store for the past 33. If I just sat down and thought about it, I could write the whole book!

So, I sat down and thought about it—and then thought about it some more. Not one memorable incident came to mind. I began to question my memory. I *am* 64, after all, and senior moments are not uncharted territory for me. But the more I thought, the more I realized that, no, nothing really monumental *has* ever happened. How could I have toiled for so many years without one life-defining, remarkable event?

Then it dawned on me: I'm a community pharmacist, not Mother Teresa! I read prescriptions and dispense drugs—period. That's what community pharmacists do. We supply sick people with medicine. We answer their questions. We get them on their way. Doing our job is not supposed to win humanitarian prizes or book awards.

So, what is it about us that *is* noteworthy? I've gathered a few suggestions.

Besides the normal prescription advice, people come to us to ask what might seem like not very monumental questions: "My 2-year-old is constipated. Do you have anything for that?" or "Tommy's got a cough. What can I give him?" or "Could you look at Jenny's rash? I have no idea what's causing it." These questions should not be answered without serious consideration. A tummy ache, a cough, a rash—all can be symptoms of more complicated conditions.

Mom didn't haul her kids out of the house, strap them into a car, and cart them to your store to get a slapdash, cavalier answer. She *especially* did not come to hear a high school clerk's opinion, no matter how many times your employee has heard the same question and knows exactly what you would say. People come to the pharmacy to talk to *you* and to get *your* advice.

They also come because your store is conveniently located (near their home with plenty of parking), you are approachable (no appointments necessary), and your advice is not only based on a college education and years of experience, but *free*. What a value! Moreover, they don't even have to wait their turn. (How many times have you had a dozen people standing at the cash register or sitting in the waiting area, one phone cradled to your ear with another one ringing, when someone walks right up and says, "If you're not too busy, could you take a look at my foot?")

Also, whatever ails them, ails them *now*. If they did call their doctor, it would be a month before they would be seen. "I'll be dead by then," they say. How many of you have heard that? So, if a person's condition really is serious, your experienced advice will send them directly to the emergency room. In that event, you really are a lifesaver.

And it's not just your community that you serve. Take for instance the elderly, out-of-town man who needs just enough digoxin to get him home. We provide it gladly—without charge.

But, doesn't it just grind you when a person brings in an empty bottle with a mail-order label and tells you that his pills are late? That person, who was once your customer, needs two Coregs until Monday. Surely, it would take more time to call the doctor, input the insurance, and process a "lost" override than to just give him two pills for free.

Here's another intangible we overlook: our ubiquitous presence in the community. Pharmacists, besides the 40-plus hours in the store, show up as city council members, Rotarians, Little League umpires, and church elders—just to name a few. We are committed people. I don't know why. It's not like it's in the job description. We are dedicated to those we serve—and in more ways than one. And this, I can assure you, doesn't go unnoticed.

Here's an example: the one personal story that finally came to me. A month ago, I went into a vacuum repair shop. I vaguely recognized the guy behind the counter but couldn't put a name to the face. Instantly, however, he recognized me. "You're Mr. Lytle, the owner of the drugstore downtown."

I answered, "That's right."

"I'll never forget you," he said. "It was 15 years ago. I fell from a ladder and screwed up my back. I was in the hospital for a month. When I got out, I was put on Vicodin. I had been on it for a few months when one day my car got broken into and my pills were stolen. I went to my regular store—a big chain near my house—and told them what happened. The guy looked at me as if to say, 'Right.' It was late Friday. He said the doctor's office was closed, and he couldn't do anything about my problem.

"As I drove past your store, I remembered meeting you somewhere—ball game, PTA, or something—so I parked and went in. I told you my problem. You called the doctor's answering service, the doctor gave you permission to give me a dozen pills, and I left. I'll never forget that. You could have turned me away, but you didn't. I started coming to you regularly, passing several other stores to get there, for over a year. Eventually, my back got better, so I haven't seen you since. I never thanked you for how you treated me when I was down."

All right, that's not exactly the "Local Pharmacist Wins Humanitarian-of-the-Year Award" story, but I bet every community pharmacist in this country has dozens, maybe thousands, of customers who, if asked to express their feelings about him or her or relate a personal story, would characterize their local pharmacist in similar glowing terms. It is why our towns need local pharmacists not only to be the first-line health care professionals, but also to do much more than that. They serve their communities, and they do it in more ways than most people imagine. •

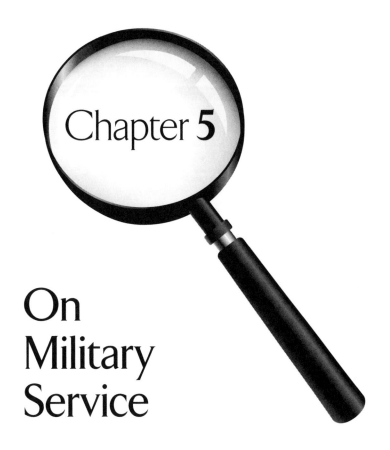

Chapter 5

On Military Service

Water, air, and cleanness are the chief articles in my pharmacy.

—Napoleon Bonaparte

It's a Small World

Patrick Garman, PharmD, PhD

Part of my job as the only clinician in an Army medical logistics unit in the run-up to Operation Iraqi Freedom was to ensure that very specialized biodefense medical products made it halfway around the world to be ready and close by if needed. The mission described here is by no means unique but is representative of what I did many times over an 8-month period from August 2002 through March 2003.

The Department of Defense reinstituted its smallpox vaccine program at the end of 2002. My mission was to escort the first shipment of this very important and very high-profile vaccine into the central command area of operations. It had to be present in each of the countries where American service members were assigned so when the order to start vaccinations was given, the program could start right away.

Military transportation was full from shuffling people, weapons systems, and other items that were needed for the coming operation. I used commercial transportation. I got to sit in the cockpit of a well-known commercial jet, with boxes of smallpox vaccine in the cargo hold. After several stops for airplane transfers and countless inventory audits on the way, I landed in one piece in the country of Qatar, where an Army medical logistics unit had set up shop to provide medical supplies to the theater.

As I disembarked from the plane and watched as my precious cargo was unloaded and then loaded onto a pallet, I began to notice the presence of "airport minders," men patrolling the runways and warehouses with small automatic weapons slung over their shoulders. As I walked behind my cargo pallet of vaccine, one of them stepped between me and the pallet just as it was about to enter the warehouse. He pointed left as my pallet was headed right. I motioned to him that I was going to follow the pallet, and he put one hand on the butt of his weapon and pointed again to the left. I went left.

I entered the airport warehouse and could see my pallet being towed into a metal cage on the other side and parked. As I stood there in 120°F heat, watching my temperature-sensitive vaccine being quarantined, I noticed one man wearing the flowing robes and headdress of a Middle Eastern sheik and sitting in an enclosed air-conditioned glass office to one side. It didn't take long to find out that he was in charge of the warehouse operation. I was not allowed to speak to him or enter his office. One of his employees came over to me after speaking to the man and said that because my shipment was medically related, it must be impounded until the Ministry of Health released it. I asked how long it would take. "Maybe a week," was the reply. My vaccine was packed to last for up to 3 to 5 days depending on ambient temperature, and I was already on day two.

As I stood looking at my career—I mean my cargo—a mere 50 yards away, thoughts of calling the local U.S. military base or calling back to the United States to ask for help were working their way through my brain. It was about that time that an unassuming man wearing several cell phones and brandishing a bright and cheerful smile approached me and said that he could help. Seems he was a Pakistani who worked as a go-between for the U.S. military and Qatari government. He worked for the commercial shipping company that had just brought me to this warehouse in Doha. He spoke very quickly but with a perfect English accent. I felt as if I was talking to my local used-car salesman as he described a network of his friends that could schedule a meeting with the Ministry of Health official that had the power to remove the quarantine on the vaccine.

My choices were limited, so I agreed to work with him. Miraculously (sarcasm intended), the official had time to see me that same day. For a small token amount of $50, my new friend could drive me to the official's office, which was on the other side of Doha. He explained that the money was for the trouble of setting up such a quick visit. So, with a newly stamped passport, the vaccine shipment's bill of lading, and $50 lighter in the wallet, I accompanied him to the Qatari Ministry of Health.

About 15 roundabouts later, we arrived at an imposing set of governmental buildings. We were let into the center parking area and escorted up to a corner set of several offices. As I entered the first room, several assistants guided me to my waiting room until the official was ready to see me. About 5 minutes later, I was told that I could see the official but my traveling friend was not allowed to go with me. As I entered the official's office, I was overwhelmed with the feeling that I had been in this room before. It reminded me of Greg Brady's room in the episode of the *Brady Bunch* when Greg attempted to turn his dad's office into his own swinging bachelor pad. There was shag carpet; fuzzy lampshades; and a weird, almost plaid, furniture design.

The man on the other side of the desk from me had very short hair and round blue glasses pushed to the end of his nose. Picture Paul Shaffer from the *Late Show with David Letterman*. He smiled and offered me some chicory tea. When I said yes, some was brought to me by one of his assistants, who lined the office.

The tea tasted like tree bark, but I obliged by sipping it along with my host. The first question the man asked me was whether I had ever been to the U.S. West Coast. In fact, my first assignment in the Army was in Southern California. We proceeded to discuss California and the various beach towns between Los Angeles and San Diego. We quickly discovered that we both liked surfing and had learned in California. The man had received his undergraduate degree at one of the California universities and had learned to surf while there. We talked at length about various surfing hotspots and in detail about the breaks at each location. He was a longboarder, as was I, since I had learned to surf later in life.

After about 45 minutes of talking, one of his assistants whispered something in his ear and he remarked that he had another meeting to attend. We both stood up and shook each other's hand, and I was escorted out of the room. As I was entering the waiting room, I was handed my bill of lading from one of the assistants. There on the front in red ink was the stamp and signature of the Ministry of Health official I had just spoken with. We met for about 50 minutes and never discussed my shipment of vaccine, but in my hand was his approval to remove the vaccine from quarantine and take it to the local U.S. Army base, Camp Doha.

My traveling partner and I made our way back to the airport warehouse. He was in a particularly good mood as he asked for another $50 for the return trip. I informed him that I was tapped out and did not have that amount on me. He just smiled and said it was not a big deal and he was just glad that everything was working out.

Upon arriving back at the warehouse, my bill of lading was taken to the well-dressed man in the air-conditioned glass office, where orders were issued to wheel my pallet out to the loading dock. I had called Camp Doha while driving back to the airport, and a contingent of soldiers from the medical logistics unit was waiting there at the loading dock with a military truck. We loaded the vaccine onto the truck and left for the base. The battery-powered refrigerated vaccine containers were safely connected to the medical logistics unit's power supply in a couple of hours, and the first part of the trip was a success. From touchdown in Qatar to arrival on base took only about 5 hours, but those 5 hours were some of the most anxious, confusing, eccentric, and exhilarating moments of my life.

This is the story of how the initial shipment of smallpox vaccine ended up in the right location to begin the Department of Defense's vaccination program in Southeast Asia, and it only cost this pharmacist 50 bucks. •

Not Just a Job

Robert DeChristoforo, MS, FASHP

My fourth and last duty station as a commissioned officer in the U.S. Public Health Service (PHS) brought me in 1979 to the National Institutes of Health (NIH) in Bethesda, Maryland. The beautiful 300-acre, college-like NIH campus is across the street from the National Naval Medical Center and several miles from the Walter Reed Army Medical Center. Nearby are the headquarters of the Food and Drug Administration, the United States Pharmacopeia, the American Pharmacists Association, and, of course, the American Society of Health-System Pharmacists. Not far away is Andrews Air Force Base.

It is well-known that NIH awards research grants; not as well-known is that it also has a federally funded research hospital under the direction of PHS and the Department of Health and Human Services. Thought by some to be a "pearl" within the federal government, NIH's Clinical Center offers researchers the opportunity to combine basic science with clinical research. "Bench to bedside" is an accurate description of the opportunity provided to investigators in the intramural research program, generally involving Phase I and early Phase II clinical trials. NIH also offers a fellowship training program for budding investigators, mentored by experts and free from many of the hassles of grant competition, insurance reimbursement, and pharmaceutical company funding. Approximately 10 percent of NIH's budget is devoted to intramural research.

The most moving and emotional aspect of my job is working with our research participants, who in some cases look to NIH as their last hope for a cure. Let me make it perfectly clear, however, that all participants are clearly told in the informed-consent process that they might not benefit from enrollment in a research protocol. Many also realize that they may be helping others in the future, even if the study will not help them in the short term. There certainly is no shortage of altruism in the halls of NIH's Clinical Center.

What has moved me the most has been seeing the children at NIH. With two daughters of my own, I have found it heartbreaking to see children with dwarfism or some other genetic defect, such as osteogenesis imperfecta. Yet despite their wheelchairs, crutches, or leg braces, the young patients smile and laugh as if

Reprinted with permission from the *American Journal of Health-System Pharmacy* (2007;64:1651–3).

nothing is wrong. Their parents are also pillars of strength. And then there are the children with cancer, who show the effects of chemotherapy and are connected to multiple IV lines but act as happy as could be. It is some consolation that some forms of childhood cancer can be cured. While thinking about how fortunate I am to have been blessed with two wonderful healthy daughters, I cannot forget that a devastating disease could strike at any time.

And then there are the children infected with HIV. HIV infection manifests itself differently in children, progressing to AIDS and death far more quickly than in adults. But first, a bit of history about the disease. Younger pharmacists may not realize that the virus that causes HIV infection and ultimately AIDS was not initially known to the medical community. In fact, it was not even known that the causative agent was a virus. In the early 1980s, NIH was an instrumental research facility for studying the disease initially known as GRID: Gay-Related Immune Deficiency. Ultimately, NIH researchers and French researchers codiscovered the "AIDS virus," which was eventually named human immunodeficiency virus, or HIV. Once the agent was discovered and the routes of transmission understood, the transmission rate could be reduced, especially to children with hemophilia who required transfusions with blood-derived products. In fact, an NIH researcher was the first to develop a test to screen blood products to stop this type of transmission. But there were no drugs to treat this new viral infection until the development of zidovudine, then known as azidothymidine, or AZT. Although initially developed with NIH grant funding as a type of cancer chemotherapy, zidovudine had been tucked away with no useful indication until testing was done at NIH for anti-HIV activity. The first patient to receive zidovudine was at the Clinical Center in a Phase I trial.

Researchers at the National Cancer Institute took zidovudine one step further by administering an investigational injectable form of the drug as a continuous infusion using ambulatory care pumps. Where else but NIH could children and their parents receive a $5,000 infusion pump (with 24-hour medical, nursing, and pharmacy support) to take home to any part of the country? There were no constraints with reimbursement—just the best possible research. This research led to a dramatic reversal of AIDS-related neurologic deterioration in these children, who soon recovered major developmental milestones, including walking, speaking, and reading, all of which had been severely impaired by the ravages of HIV infection. Advances in the treatment of HIV and AIDS have saved an estimated 3 million life-years in the United States alone.[1]

Not every disease is as well known as HIV/AIDS or gets the same amount of public attention. One of the missions of NIH is to help patients with rare diseases. What other institution would have the resources to bring in research participants from all over the country free of charge? I was fortunate to be appointed to the institutional review board of the National Eye Institute (NEI), one of the many institutes of NIH. I quickly learned that the NEI studies were referred to as "masked" rather than "blinded." One of the researchers developed a cysteamine eye drop, which literally dissolved cystine crystals that packed the cornea in the eyes of patients with cystinosis. It was like a miracle; the study's participants had their painful condition reversed, and their vision improved as long as they used the eye drops properly. How many investigational drugs are effective in over 90 percent of patients when used properly? However, this is only part of the story. For a number of reasons, the manufacture of these eye drops is still not a viable option for pharmaceutical manufacturers. Since the NIH pharmacy is the current "manufacturer," the protocol has been kept open, allowing those treated in the study to receive their eye drops and be studied further by researchers. It is the compassion of the researchers and the organization, as well as the heartfelt thanks of those who participate in the studies, that make it so rewarding to come to work each day.

One of the things that first struck me when I came to NIH was seeing a Nobel laureate walking through the halls. I recognized him as one of the authors of a neuropharmacology text I had used in pharmacy school, and here he was on the NIH staff. Little did I know that he was just one of the first nationally known researchers and authors whom I would encounter. I am not a "warm and fuzzy" kind of guy, but I was in awe of these people and felt very fortunate to be part of the same organization.

Clinical research is not without risk, though. In the early 1990s, a promising drug called flaluridine was being studied in a multicenter trial for chronic hepatitis B. Tragically, some study participants died of liver failure and other adverse effects. Two participants required liver transplants, and others suffered reversible effects. Some participants had no adverse effects at all. The public did not get to see the effect of these developments on the dedicated researchers as we did on the NIH campus. Instead, the public saw newspaper accounts (in one case on the front page) such as "And Then the Patients Suddenly Started Dying: How NIH Missed Warning Signs in Drug Test"[2] and "Optimism May Have Led to Drug Tragedy."[3] There were several investigations, debates among ethicists, and, ultimately, lawsuits. Nonetheless, the Institute of Medicine's review concluded that the studies were justified, properly designed, and well conducted, with no evidence of negligence. Even so, hepatitis drug development ceased for 2 years.

I could cite many examples of truly remarkable successes. One is NIH's pioneering work in gene therapy, including inserting foreign genes into humans and conducting clinical studies of gene therapy for cancer. Cancer vaccines have been developed to treat metastatic melanoma, and we prepare the final injectable dosage form for the protocols in our pharmacy. Maybe not every pharmacist or technician realizes that he or she may be participating, in some small way, in the development of a cure for cancer. Wouldn't that be something great to tell one's grandchildren? And yet, a famous gene therapy researcher, who has operated on a past president of the United States, waits in line and eats in the cafeteria like everyone else. On occasion, I even say hello as we pass in the halls.

A lot has changed since I first reported to NIH. New institutes and centers have been created, such as the National Human Genome Institute, the National Center for Complementary and Alternative Medicine, the Vaccine Research Center, and the Center for Biodefense and Emerging Infectious Diseases. Severe acute respiratory syndrome, or SARS, and avian influenza are some very recognizable new areas of research. NIH also dedicated a new 234-bed hospital in 2005 to continue its important work.

I completed over 33 years of active duty in the Commissioned Corps of PHS and have been fortunate to stay on as a civil servant. I feel as if my PHS and NIH colleagues are family. Research participants, partly because of their dependence on us, have become part of this extended family. Presidents, first ladies, and other dignitaries have visited to announce new initiatives to fight diseases. The U.S. surgeon general has quarters on the NIH campus, and, over the years, I have seen many who have held that office walking or jogging on campus.

NIH belongs to all of us. Unfortunately, since the tragedy of September 11 and the threats of terrorism, visitors and researchers now need to pass through multiple levels of security, bomb detectors, and electronic card keys to access the campus. This inconvenience, however, has not dampened the spirits of anyone at NIH. In some ways, it reminds us of the importance of the work that is done here and its potential impact on world health.

To paraphrase the immortal words of Lou Gehrig,[4] I truly can say that "Today I consider myself the luckiest pharmacist on the face of this earth." •

Notes

1. Walensky RP, Paltiel AD, Losina E, et al. The survival benefits of AIDS treatment in the United States. *J Infect Dis.* 2006;194:11–9.

2. Schwartz J. And then the patients suddenly started dying: how NIH missed warning signs in drug test. *Washington Post.* 1993; September 7:A1, A8–9.

3. Schwartz J. Optimism may have led to drug tragedy. *Washington Post.* 1993; November 16:A6.

4. Official Web Site of Lou Gehrig. Farewell speech. Available at: www.lougehrig.com/about/speech.htm. Accessed April 7, 2007.

The Purple Rain

Michael P. Dunphy, RPh, MS

After I graduated from pharmacy college in 1968, my draft board sent me a letter of greeting asking me to report for induction into the U.S. Army. Away I went to Fort Dix, New Jersey, for basic training and then to Fort Dix's Walson Army Hospital as a pharmacy corpsman. (The Medical Service Corps was filled in those days, so most pharmacists went into the military as enlisted soldiers.)

About halfway through my 2-year service obligation, I was notified that the Army needed a pharmacist in Camp Eagle, Vietnam, and I was chosen. It was an assignment with the 101st Airborne Division (although I did not even like to fly). I was assigned to a medical supply depot primarily to make sure antibiotics did not escape into the black market, where they brought in a lot of money and helped the Viet Cong.

We started to downsize our unit after 6 months and had to destroy some of the medicines that were in excess, including about 50 large jars of gentian violet powder. To make sure these excess medications did not fall into enemy hands, we had to truck them to the dump and destroy them ourselves. As you can imagine, when glass jars of gentian violet are thrown into a dump and broken, the powder goes everywhere. Many Vietnamese natives frequented the dump looking for items to use or sell, and many were doing just that on that day.

I did not think anything about our destruction of gentian violet until I returned to our base camp and took a shower. Suddenly, my entire body turned purple. I can only imagine the alarm that the Vietnamese dump dwellers felt when they took their next shower or their surprise the next time it rained at the dump, creating a river of purple. ●

Just Another Old Guy

Pamela Stewart-Kuhn, RPh, MPA, CGP

Being a military pharmacist has been an eye-opening experience. I'm in my 40s now, and I find that some of the new recruits weren't even born when I had already graduated from pharmacy school. There's nothing like a 20-year-old to make you realize how fast the time is passing by. With youth comes arrogance, and I was certainly not any different at the same tender age as some of my corpsmen.

What I have noticed is that the young perceive that old people have always been old. Somehow it seems inconceivable to them that the old man at the pharmacy window was once as young as they are now. They couldn't possibly have had an interesting life filled with adventure, valor, and trauma. They must have simply sprung from their mother's womb as a 70-year-old person.

I've encouraged my staff to be patient with the old guys as they rattle off their stories—they may just learn some remarkable things. Wrapped up inside those withering bodies and graying heads are some extraordinary tales.

I remember the two "old guys" that worked together on base as facilities employees, replacing lightbulbs and tightening door hinges. They had known each other since the Korean War, when they had found themselves in the same prisoner of war camp. Together, they survived, and that shared bond continued for more than 40 years. Then there was Larry, the surprisingly tall and lanky old guy, who was one of the first Navy pilots to land a plane on the deck of an aircraft carrier. I never did figure out how he could squeeze all of his height into the cockpit. There was Sarge, who despite having a body being crippled with Paget's disease, can still speak six languages, including Greek, Korean, and Farsi. He clearly remembers all of his tours of duty over a 30-year period. There was John, who was at the U.S. Embassy in Beirut shortly after it was bombed. There is the Medal of Honor recipient, one of those few who didn't receive it posthumously. There was a survivor of the Bataan Death March. There's the Navy chaplain, who has more combat ribbons than most people can identify, after serving three tours in Vietnam as a young Marine. There are many others (although their numbers are getting smaller each day) who can recall chasing Rommel across the deserts of North Africa, storming the beaches at D-Day, or fighting in the battles of Iwo Jima and Okinawa.

I've learned not to make assumptions based on what I see when another "old guy" comes up to my pharmacy window. ●

Commander Sweetie

Pamela Stewart-Kuhn, RPh, MPA, CGP

I am a Yankee, having been born and raised in the suburbs of New Jersey. As fate would have it, my military career has taken me progressively further into the South. My current duty station is in the Deep South, so far south in Alabama that the next stop is the Gulf of Mexico. I've grown to like the South, and I enjoy the warm climate and Southern hospitality. I've gotten used to little old ladies and Southern gentlemen calling me "sugar," "honey," and "sweetie" in places such as church or the local diner. I'm also a female pharmacist, which isn't so out of the ordinary in 2008. I've enjoyed a respectable level of success in my career, and with 18 years of service, I hold the rank of commander.

Many of the patients that come to my pharmacy are retired. Most of them retired long before women in the military enjoyed an equal status with their male counterparts. To many, a female commander is an anomaly. I work in a climate where respect, equality, and "politically correct" language are expected by all members of the service.

A couple of years ago, I received a new pharmacy technician fresh out of school and in her very early 20s. She grew up in the Midwest and in the more modern climate of women's rights. When one of the retirees came in one day and greeted me with "Hi, sweetie," the young technician was taken aback. I explained that we were in the Deep South, and I didn't take the endearment as offensive or derogatory.

"Still," she told me adamantly, "You're a commander and should not be referred to as 'sweetie.'"

A few days later, a retired master chief that I had known for several years came into my pharmacy with his characteristic, "Hi, sweetie."

I said, "Master Chief, that's Commander Sweetie to you!"

I still use that phrase, as a well-meaning joke with several of my retirees. ●

The Greatest Generation

Anita Airee, PharmD

I've been a pharmacist for 11 years and have had the privilege of caring for the generation of individuals known as "the greatest generation" of Americans. As an American-born daughter of immigrants, these extraordinary people did not grace any family reunions, so the opportunity I had to interact with them while working primarily in ambulatory care clinics across Tennessee and Florida was and continues to be the most rewarding and enriching experience of my career.

Never was this more evident than while I was working in Oak Ridge, Tennessee, also known as the "Secret City," the home of the Manhattan Project. After spending 7 years (1999–2006) working in this small city in three separate venues—hospital, clinic, and retail pharmacy—I had the distinct pleasure to meet the individuals who actually worked on the Manhattan Project, as well as those who served the city and the country through the difficult times preceding August 6, 1945. Their attitudes toward their jobs and their country were simple and absolute. They had a duty, and they performed it. (They responded to their pharmacy care in like fashion, making them easily adherent toward any intervention I made.)

The couple who led the first Oak Ridge Symphony, the individual who refuted the China Syndrome to the Department of Energy, and the women who worked within the plants would wear their identification badges on Secret City Day. These were just a few of the individuals I had the honor to meet. I heard stories from men about the muddy roads of the city and how difficult it was to "court their ladies" during this time. I talked to people who knew Albert Einstein personally. (They said he often wore the same suit with the same grease stain on the front.) People related stories to me about how the word spread on V-J Day. I had a book about the history of Oak Ridge. Many of my patients could point to themselves or people they knew on the cover, which had a photograph from the day Japan surrendered showing ecstatic individuals holding up newspapers with the "War Ends" headlines. I made them sign my book!

I spent as much time as my position would allow being a willing ear for their stories. As I spent time with these people, I witnessed the quiet strength of character from a generation that accepted sacrifice as the norm. These opportunities were rare and priceless, and I felt honored to be a firsthand listener. In a way, I felt grateful to be a pharmacist at what I felt was the perfect time, particularly in Oak Ridge, because I was able to capture these stories in their subjects' waning days.

I would often ask them what they thought of the country now. The most common response was a shake of the head and, with an air of sadness, "It is not the same." They were discouraged, yet in keeping with their character, they remained quiet about it unless probed. Although I encouraged many to get involved in the community by mentoring or serving in civic organizations, most of them seemed resigned to their current duty in life as they perceived it—not to get involved, not to interfere.

It was and still is my desire to have my pharmacy students get to know the men and women of this generation; they offer one of the most priceless educational experiences anyone could have. Perhaps the younger generation will pay tribute to this finest generation of individuals by living their example and creating another great generation. ●

Funny the Things That People Don't Notice

J. Aubrey Waddell, PharmD, FAPhA, BCOP

I spent 22 years of my pharmacy career as a U.S. Army pharmacy officer. During a career of that length, an Army pharmacy officer can expect to practice in a wide variety of settings, spanning everything from provision of pharmacy services in a combat zone to institutional clinical pharmacy practice to regulatory pharmacy practice to managerial pharmacy practice to hospital pharmacy practice to community pharmacy practice. For those of us who have done this, one of the sacred constants is 99 percent of the complaints against an Army pharmacy officer are due to something that happens at an Army community pharmacy.

The Army, like all the services, uses the chain of command as the first location of all complaints from active-duty members, active-duty family members, and retirees. However, the Army has a unique position that it uses as a place for fielding complaints that a person might not want to take to the chain of command for various reasons, such as when the complaint involves a member of the chain of command. That position is called the inspector general, or IG, and any officer or senior enlisted person might be trained and appointed as the IG for his or her command. Typically, being an IG is a full-time job in the Army. However, IGs in smaller commands (such as a small Army hospital) might do the job on an as-needed basis while also holding another full-time position. Such was my situation from 1990 to 1991, when I was assigned as chief of the pharmacy service at Patterson Army Community Hospital at Fort Monmouth, New Jersey, while also being appointed as the hospital's IG.

I quickly discovered that more than 90 percent of the complaints I fielded were against my own pharmacy. That was not really surprising, since my community pharmacy saw many, many more patients per day than any other service of the hospital. Another aspect of the IG job certainly was surprising, as I will explain.

As chief of the pharmacy service, I was frequently summoned by my staff to talk to patients who had various complaints, such as prescription waiting time, nonavailability of a prescribed medication, nonformulary drug issues, and perceived rudeness of my staff. Most of the time, I could resolve the complaint, but when I couldn't, the discussion with the patient would boil down to the patient saying something like, "That's it. I can see you can't help me. I want to speak to the hospital IG."

At this point, I would tell the person in front of me, "That's fine sir/ma'am. Just walk down that hallway, go to the next intersection, take another right, and then enter the next door on the right. You'll see a waiting area there that leads into an office. That's the IG's office, and if you will knock on that door, the IG will invite you in and take care of your complaint." While the patient was winding around the hallways that surrounded the pharmacy, I would go to my office and sit down and wait. In a couple of minutes, there would be a knock on the door. I would politely invite the patient in, carefully record the complaint, and assure the patient that I would call him or her soon with a resolution.

The surprising thing is, in 2 years of doing that, not a single patient ever noticed that the pharmacy chief and the IG were in fact *the same person*. The patients talked about the pharmacy chief in the second person, even using my name and rank, and I would dutifully write down everything they said, all the while sitting there wearing a uniform that boldly proclaimed the same name and rank! Pursuant to my IG oath, I always thoroughly investigated every complaint and always called the patients with their expected resolutions, as though I were two people. It was surreal. If resolution of the complaint dictated that I have a meeting with the pharmacy chief, then I would simply talk to myself about the problem and come to a resolution.

Ever since that experience, I have made a special effort to really *notice* people with whom I interact, no matter what the situation. •

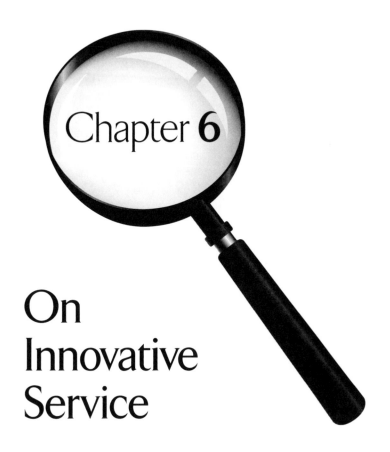

Chapter 6

On Innovative Service

Just a spoonful of sugar helps the medicine go down.

—Richard M. Sherman and
Robert B. Sherman, *songwriters*

Interventions Notably Improve
Patient Treatment

Submitted by the Koninklijke Nederlandse Maatschappij ter bevordering der Pharmacie (Royal Dutch Association for the Advancement of Pharmacy)

R esearch has indicated that nearly 15 percent of hospital intakes for gastro-intestinal bleeding can be prevented. Three pharmacists in the Netherlands decided to do something about it. They now give gastroprotection to patients who use a certain combination of medicines, and they are proud they can help their patients in this way.

HARM Study
A group of 14 general pharmacists and hospital pharmacists in the Brabant region have joined together to form the Brabant Institute for Pharmacy Research, or BIRD. Every year, BIRD members select a topic for further investigation. The focus is always on practicality and health care benefit.

Inge Coehorst works as a pharmacist for the Blaak and Zorgvlied pharmacies in the city of Tilburg and has been a BIRD member for several years. Inge says, "When we got together in 2006, the HARM [Hospital Admissions Related to Medication] study had just been publicized.[1] The HARM results showed that 46 percent of hospital admissions in the Netherlands were related to medication—14.5 percent were caused by gastrointestinal bleeding occurring as a result of certain combinations of medicines. Had these patients received gastroprotection, their hospitalization could have potentially been avoided. We decided to focus on this particular subject."

Results Shocked Pharmacists
Inge, together with two other pharmacists, took the lead in drawing up a plan and carrying it out. To start with, they wanted to know what the situation in the Brabant region was really like. From October 2006 to April 2007, they performed a baseline measurement. They checked the systems of participating pharmacies for instances when gastroprotection was given to patients who used a combination of a nonsteroidal anti-inflammatory drug (NSAID) and aspirin. Their colleagues were surprised: "Of course we give these patients gastroprotection!" However, the research showed otherwise—59 percent of the target group did not receive gastroprotective medication.

Inge recalls, "That really came as a shock. And immediately the question arose of how could this have happened." The staggeringly high percentage proved to be the result of a combination of factors: guidelines that were too vague, doctors who were insufficiently aware that low-dosage or short use of NSAIDs can cause problems, and doctors who were reluctant to prescribe yet another tablet for the patient. The conclusion on the basis of first-time dispensing was clear: Methods had to be improved. The next step was to inform the doctors in the region and come to an agreement on how to proceed.

Cooperation with Doctors

The three pharmacists prepared a standard presentation about the HARM study and the results from the baseline measurement in the participating pharmacies. All BIRD pharmacists gave this presentation during regular professional meetings with doctors. Nearly all the doctors were fully convinced and indicated that they would start to prescribe a gastroprotective in the case of an NSAID and aspirin combination.

In October 2007, BIRD pharmacists and participating doctors began using these new guidelines. Inge states, "Because of our excellent relationship with the doctors, we were able to come to an agreement to take the procedure a couple of steps further. Pharmacists were to alert the doctors when they forgot to prescribe gastroprotection. And, in case the doctor could not be reached, the pharmacist was to add the gastroprotective to the prescription. The doctor would be contacted later and asked to alter the prescription. It was quite something that we were able to convince the doctors to work in this way."

Simple Procedure, Great Effect

The goal was simple: After 6 months, 90 percent of the patients should have received the correct treatment. In April 2008, another measurement was taken. The original baseline of 59 percent had dropped to 32 percent. This meant that 68 percent of patients were treated according to the new guidelines. Inge says, "I admit we did not reach our goal, but we have in the meantime figured out the principal reason why. The medical specialists and dentists had not been asked to participate. Now, they too follow the new procedure. But, in any case, we did manage to convince everyone that our active interventions have brought about a notable improvement in patient treatment. There is now a 2.7-fold better chance that a patient who uses the combination of an NSAID and aspirin will receive proper gastroprotection medication."

All the pharmacists and pharmacy assistants involved are fully trained to watch out for this medicine combination. Every day, they check medication regimens and call the doctors if necessary. Inge says enthusiastically, "It has really become a standard daily practice in our pharmacies. The good thing is that such a simple pharmacy procedure can so much improve the well-being of our patients. At the same time, it highlights our added value as pharmacists and greatly improves our contacts with the doctors. We are rather proud of our achievement."

And rightly so. In 2009, the Koninklijke Nederlandse Maatschappij ter bevordering der Pharmacie (Royal Dutch Association for the Advancement of Pharmacy) selected this project for the annual Pharmaceutical Care Awards. ●

Note

1. Leendertse AJ, Egberts AC, Stoker JL, Van den Bemt PM: HARM Study Group. Frequency of and risk factors for preventable medication-related hospital admissions in the Netherlands. *Arch Intern Med.* 2008;168(17):1890–6.

A Bridge Between Hospital and Patients

Submitted by the Koninklijke Nederlandse Maatschappij ter bevordering der Pharmacie (Royal Dutch Association for the Advancement of Pharmacy)

Project developed by Nora Zoet and Arjan Groote

More control, increased adherence, and improved monitoring of medication and patient care are the results of close cooperation between our pharmacy, the 24-hour Waterland Pharmacy in Purmerend, and the city's family doctors, medical specialists, and nurses.

For some time, doctors at the Waterland Hospital and pharmacists from the Waterland Pharmacy had pondered the idea of shifting certain kinds of pharmaceutical care away from the hospital to the patient's home. So, when our plan was proposed, the climate was right.

Epoetin Administered at Home

We began with the patient group that was prescribed epoetin 1 month before planned orthopedic surgery. Usually, these patients had to visit the hospital four times to receive their epoetin injections. Some doctors had already informed us that these patients could just as well receive the treatment at home. We then took the lead and organized a meeting with the doctors and nurses. Together, we determined a course of action, and in spring 2008, we started administering at home. We have worked in this way for a year now, and all the health care professionals involved are happy with the results of this new approach. It also saves our patients a lot of hassle, so they approve too.

Helps Reduce Stress

The home administration of epoetin starts when patients enter the hospital 1 month before the operation. They meet one of the two hospital nurses, who are hired by the pharmacy. The nurses will later visit them at home and schedule the visits. Then, the patients visit the pharmacy, which is located in the hospital building. The pharmacist immediately coordinates the process and contacts the orthopedic surgeon if necessary. The lines of communication are very short, reducing the risk of misunderstanding.

Our new method of working has created a bridge between hospital and patient. The patient receives high-quality specialist care in the comfort of his or her home. An operation always causes a great deal of anxiety, and this program helps reduce that stress. The program is especially helpful for elderly and less mobile patients. Additionally, the home is a more relaxed environment in which to explain the operation.

Gonadotropin-Releasing Hormone Analogs

Similar procedures have already been discussed with gynecologists and urologists for patient treatment with gonadotropin-releasing hormone analogs because these drugs need to be administered regularly. We have arranged for these specialists to access a protected page in the pharmacy's Web site. Reminders alert the pharmacists when patients are scheduled to receive injections. The pharmacists in turn notify the nurses, who make appointments for home visits. If a patient prefers that a family doctor administer the injection, that too can be arranged. Thus, the patient has a say in the matter and feels more in control of the situation. Additionally, we hope this cooperation will be broadened to include other specialties.

Optimal Adherence

The medical specialists are able to monitor medication use via computer. When, for example, doctors find an unexpected laboratory value, they can be sure it is not the result of incorrect use of medication. Additionally, our pharmacy is connected to the computer system of the general pharmacies in town, ensuring that we always have a complete overview of a patient's medication.

We have achieved what we had hoped for: optimal adherence and high-quality pharmaceutical care. In 2009, the Koninklijke Nederlandse Maatschappij ter bevordering der Pharmacie (Royal Dutch Association for the Advancement of Pharmacy) selected this project for the annual Pharmaceutical Care Awards. ●

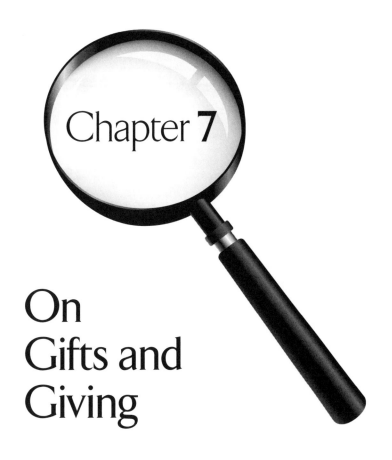

Chapter 7

On
Gifts and
Giving

The greatest gift is a portion of thyself.

—Ralph Waldo Emerson

I Hope You Like Country Music

Heather Eppert, PharmD, BCPS

I was working at a rural health clinic, and one of the physicians came into my office and shut the door. The physician informed me that he had two patients, husband and wife, who had recently suffered a great deal of loss, both personally and financially, and that they were going to need assistance obtaining their medications. However, the husband was a very proud farmer, and he refused to sign up for any public assistance programs. The physician asked me to speak with the husband and wife. I spoke at length with the couple regarding various treatment options, and finally, they were willing to apply for assistance through several of the pharmaceutical manufacturers.

About 8 weeks later, all the medications had arrived. The couple was in such a poor financial situation that they easily qualified for the patient assistance programs. I packaged the medications and called the couple to inform them that the medications were ready to pick up. The husband told me that they would be coming to town the next day for a few things and would swing by the office on their way to town. I said that I would not be in the office in the morning but would leave the medications in a secure location. The physician could help them. I hung up the telephone and didn't think anymore about it.

I arrived in my office the next day to find a small package on my desk with a little note on the outside, written in the penmanship of an old farmer. The note read, "I know that I am a proud man, and I don't have much, but I sure thank you for your hard work. I hope you like country music." It closed with his signature. In the package, wrapped in a small brown paper bag that had been cut up, was a cassette tape. On the outside of the cassette was his name, the date, and "Thank You." I placed the cassette in a player, and to my amazement, it was the farmer playing his guitar and singing some famous old country tunes. The mere thought of the situation brought tears to my eyes.

He has long since passed on. However, I still have the tape, and I play it from time to time. To this day, this gift remains one of the most heartfelt, caring ones that I have ever received. That proud old farmer didn't have "anything" to give me that day, so he put his pride to the side and gave me a small piece of himself. ●

A Gift of Inspiration

Jessica Stovel, Hon BSc, BScPhm

I t was the beginning of summer and the end of residency. At long last, I was about to embark upon my career as a pharmacist. I was starting my first week of my future clinical area: pediatric hematology/oncology. After attending rounds on my new service, the training pharmacist assigned me my first patient, a 9-year-old girl who had just been diagnosed with Ewing's sarcoma. I reviewed her chart and prepared to do a medication history. With a combination of nervous anticipation and hesitancy over what to expect, I looked forward to applying in practice the pharmaceutical care model that I learned throughout university and my hospital residency. I was hoping that I could in some way positively affect and improve the care of this child. Little did I imagine at the time that she would so profoundly affect and shape me, both professionally and personally.

Even though her care eventually transferred to another pharmacist, I continued to follow her closely over the next 7 months—and helped where I could with the many drug-related issues that arose. Having a particularly difficult time with each round of chemotherapy and then radiation, this little angel of a girl went through what seemed to be an unending stream of neuropathic pain to the point where she could no longer walk unassisted. She bravely endured intense and frequent nausea, vomiting, and a host of other traumatic treatment-related adverse effects too numerous to list. What continuously amazed me was her constant optimism about her life, her family, and her future. Moreover, no matter what trials she was forced to suffer or how horrible a day she was having, she always gave me a smile, a wave, and a "thank you."

My spirits were always lifted when I saw her because she reminded me to have a positive outlook and not to take a single second for granted. Through her dignity and stoicism, I learned the definition of true strength, courage, and perseverance. I watched with awe as she faced terrible and seemingly endless challenges. No matter how emotionally distressing these experiences must have been inwardly, outwardly, she maintained a positive and confident attitude. She was determined to be strong, not only for herself, but also for those around her. The indomitable spirit of this remarkable girl has changed me profoundly. I have gained new perspectives on life, bravery, and the courage to face adversity.

Complete selflessness also comes to mind when I think about her. I will never forget Christmas Eve, when she unexpectedly required an overnight admission. I knew she had been so looking forward to spending Christmas at home with her family and would be desperately disappointed at this setback. Nevertheless, when I visited her that evening, she was less concerned about her own needs than learning what I wanted from Santa for Christmas. This moment was yet another that utterly touched me. This innocent child focused completely on my happiness at Christmastime, when she must have been distraught at missing the holiday traditions she longed to share with her big sister and parents.

Beyond affecting me personally, she has also taught me much about the practitioner that I want to be. Not only did the suffering she had to endure reinforce the importance of providing patient-centered care, but also the complexity of her condition and medications taught me the value of continuity of care as patients transition between the inpatient and outpatient worlds. I learned that developing a seamless process of communication between outpatient clinics and community pharmacies, as well as conducting consistent medication reconciliation and reassessment processes upon readmission as an inpatient, ensured best patient outcomes. This experience showed me how valuable such services could be and helped me see how I wanted to practice as a pharmacist on that service. Moreover, as a new pharmacist with many obstacles to overcome in establishing my practice, my first patient will always remind me why I do what I do and why it is worth it. She is a constant inspiration.

In addition to being shaped by her, I was also deeply touched by the love and devotion of her family. Her older sister worked and studied exceptionally hard throughout the 7 months, even though she was constantly separated from her mother and sister because the hospital was 2 hours away from their home. She continued to obtain high marks in all her high school classes, despite the tremendous stress and worry she had to bear. Again, this perseverance in the face of adversity was inspirational to me. More important, their caring relationship taught me to understand the strength of bonds that can exist between sisters. As an only child, I was moved to see how close the girls were and how they supported each other. The little sister's one wish on that Christmas Eve was to have her older sister with her in the hospital so that she could read her their traditional story.

The parents were also incredibly dedicated and caring. Their daughter was never left alone. Her mother was at her bedside throughout each night she was in the hospital. I recall several occasions when her mother would not even take a break to get a snack, because she didn't want to leave her daughter. I know what a profound difference this made and understood where her daughter derived much of her strength. Her father was also an inspiration to me because he traveled the

2-hour trip to the hospital every weekend and often multiple times a week. He did this while maintaining his job, caring for his older daughter, and being the family's rock of support. Both parents were so brave throughout the ordeal and worked hard to maintain a positive and optimistic environment for their daughter.

My many interactions with the entire family on both a professional and personal level taught me the true meaning of strength, unity, love, and sacrifice. This family also showed me what a difference such hope, faith, and belief can make. The little girl has made it through her several courses of chemotherapy and radiation, returned home to her family and new puppy, and emerged an even stronger girl than she was initially. I have been forever changed by this special angel and her devoted family. ●

Coumadin Clinic Encounters

Jason Hutchens, PharmD

I am a clinical pharmacist at a community hospital in Maryville, Tennessee. I mainly provide inpatient clinical services, but I am also the coordinator for the outpatient Coumadin clinic that serves approximately 300 patients. I have been seeing some of the Coumadin patients for several years, so often visits include time catching up on how the family is doing and other small talk. I have had many meaningful encounters throughout the years, but three recent events stick out in my mind.

The first involved an elderly woman brought in by her daughter, who was about 60 years old, and their female neighbor with a newborn baby. As they pulled into the parking lot, a tire on their car went flat. They came in for the appointment and told me about the tire and that they had called the neighbor's husband to come to their rescue. The problem was that he was going to drive about 30 miles just to change a flat tire. I told the women that if they would give me a couple of minutes to catch up on the patients who were in the waiting room, I would be happy to change the tire. So, in my dress shirt and slacks, I found myself in the parking lot with grease on my hands and head. The women were extremely thankful and to this day sing my praises.

The second involved another elderly woman whose complete blood count showed she was very anemic. After I questioned her about any bleeding that she was experiencing, she finally admitted to me that she had some bloody stools. She became emotional and teary-eyed, explaining to me that the health care system was confusing and intimidating. She asked for a hug, telling me that she felt scared and alone. She further explained that she felt like I was the only one she could turn to whom she could trust and who really cared. I obliged her with the requested hug and calmed her down. I explained that she needed to go straight to the emergency room and that she would likely be admitted for a blood transfusion and some gastrointestinal testing to find the source of her blood loss. I saw her the next day in the hospital, and she was very grateful that I took the time to explain the situation to her and the steps she needed to take to resolve it.

The third encounter happened while I was making rounds in the hospital. The son of one Coumadin clinic patient recognized me while I was sitting in one of our units. The patient had just had surgery, and the family was visiting. He came over to me and said, "Could you step in and see my mother for a minute? It would really mean a lot to her." Of course, I said sure and went in to talk to the nice elderly woman. She had had an extensive surgery and was still waiting for the nurse to give her some pain medication. When I walked in, I greeted her and asked how she was feeling. She replied, "I feel better now that you are here. I always look forward to seeing you."

The moral of these stories: A little compassion and a caring attitude are our best medicine. ●

Insulin Syringes and a Young Marine Wife

J. Aubrey Waddell, PharmD, FAPhA, BCOP

In the mid-1980s, I was running the pharmacy in the U.S. Army Health Clinic at Yuma Proving Ground, Arizona, a remote post more than 30 miles from the city of Yuma. "Running the pharmacy" is a bit of an overstatement—I was the only pharmacist, and I had one Army pharmacy technician.

The great majority of my patients were active-duty or family-member residents of the post or military retirees from nearby RV parks, but one day a very young woman from the city of Yuma showed up at my pharmacy window. She asked whether I had the "new" insulin syringes, which had a higher-gauge needle—28 gauge I believe—rather than the usual 26-gauge needles. The higher-gauge needles were less painful to use. I told her that I did have the syringes and would be happy to dispense them to her every month with a prescription from her physician, as our regulations then required.

Her reaction was not what I expected—she looked downcast. After a few moments of silence, she asked whether our clinic could provide a supply of these syringes each month to her clinic at Marine Corps Air Station Yuma. I told her that was probably not possible, and I asked her why she wanted to know. She hesitated and then told me that she and her Marine husband had only one vehicle. They lived on the other end of town from the air station, and he had to drive the vehicle to work each day for a variety of logistical reasons. She quickly added that this was not a burden to her, because everything she needed was within walking distance, and because she had diabetes, the daily walking was important anyway.

Her only wish, she said, was that she could get the new syringes so that her daily insulin injections wouldn't be so painful. The clinic on her base did not have the new ones in stock yet, and it would be some time before it did. (Although this may seem strange to nonmilitary types, it probably seems perfectly normal to anyone who tried to navigate the military's medical supply system in the 1980s.) I didn't have to ask why she didn't buy them at a local pharmacy, because I knew that a young Marine's income would not allow for purchasing medical supplies outside of those provided free of charge by the base clinic. I took her prescription and gave her a month's supply of the syringes. She thanked me and left. I never did figure out how she got all the way out to my clinic on that day. I couldn't stop thinking about her predicament as I walked home.

That night, when I told my wife of the experience, she looked at me strangely (as she often does when my brain's logic centers are failing me) and asked why I wouldn't take the syringes to the woman each month. I replied that that would be unusual, but then she reminded me that I visited that base 2 nights a week anyway because I was taking graduate courses in business administration at their education center. Surely, she asked, couldn't the woman and I find someplace to meet on my route once a month?

The next morning, I pulled the prescription from my files (sorry, young folks, no computers in small Army pharmacies back then) and called the phone number written on it. The young woman was delighted with my wife's idea and said that she and her husband lived just a few blocks from a corner strip mall that I passed on my way to the air station.

So, that's how it was that one night a month for the next year, I would pull into a parking space at the strip mall, a young woman would approach me, I would hand her a box of insulin syringes, she would hand me a prescription, and we would part ways. It must have looked odd to anyone who cared to notice.

The young woman stopped calling me to arrange our trade about a year later, and a quick call to her clinic pharmacy confirmed that she and her husband had moved on to their next assignment. By then, the military medical supply operation had caught up with the modern syringe world, and I doubt she had any more trouble getting the better syringes.

Now, all these 25 years later, I can't remember her name or even what she looked like. However, I do remember the wonderful feeling of knowing that I was going the extra mile to do my job—caring for those who serve our nation, sometimes in isolated and small places. ●

Hot Apple Pie

Keith A. Wagner, PharmD

A general's wife came to the outpatient pharmacy window at my U.S. Army hospital to submit a prescription for cephalexin for her sinusitis. She appeared miserable and wanted to get her medications quickly and go home. I explained to her that she would probably not feel any better after taking this antibiotic, and if she could sit down for a few minutes, I would obtain a different antibiotic that would make her feel better in 3 to 5 days. I then jokingly added that if she did feel better in 3 to 5 days, she would owe me a hot apple pie. She agreed and sat down in the waiting area.

I grabbed a prescription pad, wrote down a more effective antibiotic for sinusitis, and walked over to the appropriate hospital clinic to find the doctor who wrote the first prescription. When I found him, I told him that I thought he meant to write for this other antibiotic. He agreed and signed the prescription. I returned to the pharmacy and filled the prescription for the patient and sent her on her way.

The following week, I was talking to my boss, and one of my technicians approached us and said that a general's wife was in the pharmacy lobby with a hot apple pie for me. ●

Drugs on a Plane

Paul R. Bergeron II, RPh

I was working for the AARP pharmacy service in Long Beach, California, when I received a call from the association's travel service, located upstairs in the building we shared. A Continental Airlines jet had skidded off the runway at Los Angeles International Airport during its departure to Hawaii. About 50 AARP travel-service customers had been on board and were forced to abandon the plane using the escape chutes.

The travel service had always recommended that its members keep their prescription drugs with them in their purses or carry-on bags because luggage stowed below was subject to being lost or delayed. However, because of the unexpected departure from the plane, all the AARP members had left everything, including their prescription drugs, on board, and they could not be retrieved.

The service asked me whether I would be able to visit each family at their hotel, get a list of drugs needed and hometown pharmacy, call the pharmacy for copies, come back to the AARP pharmacy, fill the prescriptions, and return them to their members. And, could I do it right away, because they would be off to Hawaii on another flight the next day?

"Yes, yes, and yes," I responded. Because our pharmacy was a big operation, employing more than 20 pharmacists and 130 support staff, I was able to devote the next 24 hours to helping out these families.

It was the most enjoyable incident of my now 48 years in pharmacy. The people were delighted to see me. Most were watching their own exploits on TV. One gentleman was sitting in a chair with jet-fuel-soaked trousers up to his knees—smoking a cigarette! Another passenger spent 5 minutes explaining that he was "actually not old enough to be an AARP member" but was just accompanying someone who was. All were upbeat, and all had decided that this mishap would not keep them from going to Hawaii. They were also happy that I had made myself available to help them.

I was just as happy. Talk about good customer service—they could now fly to Hawaii with all of their prescription meds with them. ●

Best Steak Ever

L. Douglas Ried, PhD

Mr. Sam Patient had been coming to my pharmacy for his gout medicine and SerApEs (a combination of reserpine, hydralazine, and hydrochlorothiazide) for his high blood pressure (HBP) for more than a year. The prescription was for a 30-day supply of each, and for the longest time, he got them both on the same day. However, one day, I noticed that he was getting his gout medicine more frequently than his HBP medicine. I asked him whether he was taking his HBP medicine as directed and he said no. Sam told me that this medication was causing him a lot of side effects, so he had cut down on the amount he was taking and was feeling much better.

Sam was looking very red-faced and flushed to me, and I asked him how long it had been since he had his blood pressure checked. He said it had been several months, because he was feeling better since he started taking less of the HBP medicine. I asked, "Sam, why are you getting just one of your medications as directed by your doctor?"

"Well, Doug, whenever I take fewer gout tablets, my feet start hurting. So, I take them. The other pills make me dizzy and tired all the time."

"Sam, you had better get your blood pressure checked," I instructed.

Sam responded, "It is pretty expensive to go to the doctor, and my next appointment is in 6 months. Money's a little short, and I don't have insurance. I'll just have to wait until my next appointment."

I was worried about Sam because I knew that his blood pressure was very high before he started taking his medication. So, I said, "Sam, I'm worried about your blood pressure. I tell you what—you go to the doctor as soon as possible. If your blood pressure is normal, I'll pay for the office visit. If it is not, then we'll go out for dinner one night and you can pay for the steak."

A couple of weeks later, Sam came into the pharmacy with two new prescriptions: one for gout medication and the other for HBP medication. I asked him what had happened.

Sam said, "Well, I went to the fire station and the emergency medical technician took my blood pressure. He didn't tell me what it was but said that I needed to go see my doctor right away. So, I made an appointment. The next day, the nurse took my blood pressure. She immediately left the exam room to get the doctor. The doctor took my blood pressure. He looked at me very seriously and said, 'Sam, I am going to call an ambulance and get you to the hospital immediately.' My heart doctor met me at the hospital and put me on medications right away. Later, my regular doctor told me that my blood pressure was 240 over 150 when I was in his office and that was why he sent me to the hospital in an ambulance. He was worried that I would have a stroke right then and there!"

It was the best steak I had eaten in a long time. ●

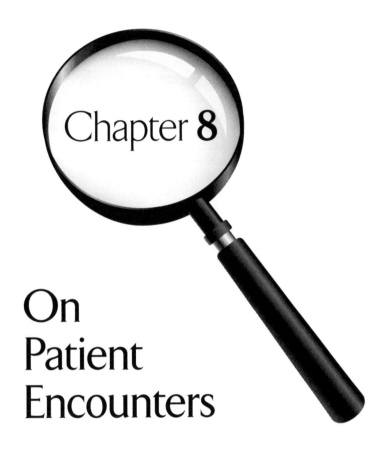

Chapter 8

On Patient Encounters

A little Consideration, a little Thought for Others, makes all the difference.

—A. A. Milne

The Magic Man

Julian Judge, MPSI, BSc(Pharm), Dip Grad Psych

Pat was the magic man. He had no address. Well, he had a few, but none that would last long enough for a file, so there was no point. His script never had a surname, just "Pat." Everything about him was average except his dress. Ties were always battered and badly knotted, but you could see the rainbow in them, such were their colours, rich and deep. He said it made them more visible, to distract the audience. His jackets were always an autumn brown, and they had more pockets than you could ever imagine. Lastly was the hat. It was like a mongrel bowler but always straight with a solid rim. It could be said it was the hat that kept him together.

At first, I didn't know how to handle a man who wouldn't give his surname. I mean, it sounds funny, but I guess everyone owns their own name and it's their choice whom to tell. It's just that it's probably the most essential and basic requirement of a prescription. There's a perception that the drugs are the key issue, but that's not necessarily the case. Sure, it's not good if you dispense the wrong drug or incorrect dosage, but the biggest mistake you will ever make is when you get the names wrong. That way, patient X gets the drugs for patient Y. You mix up those names, and you're staring at a big black hole.

Now, doctors can be contrary. You want to have good reason to call them. It's like a lucky bag: You could get juicy fruit or some sort of castrated weasel. I just about knew this doctor well enough to ring. So I did, and he wouldn't stop laughing.

"Good luck with that. I've been seeing him for a year and he won't say."

And then, "Let me know if he tells you. He knows his days of the week though. Good luck!"

I tried to reason with Pat, but it just wasn't happening. He rearranged his hat and, patting his hands on his chest, gave me his logic.

"Look, today's Tuesday. It's my favourite day and you seem like a decent fella, so I'll tell you. I'm a magician. You sell trust, and I sell illusion. Them drugs may work or not. Who knows? But above all you sell trust. Sick folks need trust, and

---

Originally published in the *Irish Pharmacist*. Adapted with permission from GreenCross Publishing.

that means needing to trust you. That's why you want their name. Well, it's the opposite I sell. The less people know or trust about me the better. I don't sell trust or fact or cures or anything like such. I sell illusion. In a way, it could be said I sell nothing. Now, young fella, do you follow me?"

One voice in my head said, "Patience." Others said different, but this was good stuff. It wasn't boring, that was for sure, plus there was something about Pat. Like a half-smile on a girl you've just met. He clapped, and a fiver floated to the counter.

"How'd you do that?"

"Oh never mind. Look, it's a simple prescription. Been getting them for years. I knew this lady down in Shannon, and she used to give me loads. Ye see, she had a medical card and let on to her quack she had asthma. I've a boat there, but she's gone now, God bless her. And that's why I'm here with you. Quack said that you'd look after me. So look, I'll just ask for the one off you. Give me the blue inhaler, and I'll give you the fiver. Now that's fair."

The morning had gone into the surreal and I knew that, but like I said he had a half-smile that just drew you in. I gave him the inhaler. He slapped the counter.

"Tickety boo! That fiver's yours now."

I'd never heard that one before. And then, "Give it back here. I want to check something."

By now, staff had gathered round. He took the note and held it up to the light as if he were saying mass, looked at me and straightening his hat, tore the fiver in two.

"Hang on," he said. "I need to test something."

He opened the inhaler and inhaled two puffs.

"That's good stuff. Just wanted to check. Now, I'll be good to you today. Watch this carefully."

He began emptying his pockets. Out came coins, pieces of coloured paper, elastic bands, tape, pieces of string—it just went on.

"Ah, here we are," he said as he pulled out the whitest handkerchief you ever saw.

"Now young fella, ask one of those lovely girls to pick up the torn fiver."

I didn't need to ask. A pair of hands grabbed it.

"Oh, now there's the girl for me. Look at those hands. Tell me, my dear, what should I call you?"

"Trish," she replied, blushing a bit.

"Well isn't that amazing. That's one of the names I call my boat. Lovely name that. Now you place those in here." Opening the handkerchief.

"That's it. Now close it and squeeze tightly! That's it Trish! Now give back."

Pat flashed his hands, and with a clap, the clean fiver floated down on the counter.

"Never give something back son. You might never see it again." Turning to Trish, he asked, "What's your friend called?'

"Helena."

"Oh Helena! I used to know someone by that name once. Girls, they're both special names. There's something ... how shall I put it? There's something magic in them. That's magic! Bye now, girls!"

This went on all summer. Every inhaler came with a new trick. The whole shop would stop, and customers and staff would watch as Pat made all sorts of things appear from his handkerchief. Children loved him, Helena began to adore him, and above all he cheered everyone up.

One morning he gave me a choice of a fiver or whatever the handkerchief would produce. A customer had a few children with her, and their open faces told me what I had to do. I got three pounds and an egg that day. Helena and Trish got a bag of bonbons.

Pat had this way about him such that even though you knew you were being robbed, you still felt that you'd got something. He'd draw you in, and you wouldn't even know it. Everybody wanted to know how the trick worked, but Pat wouldn't tell.

"If I tell you ... you won't want to know. It's like wondering if someone loves you. Take this lovely pair of beauties you have working for you here. I like to think they want me, but once I know, then the magic's gone. That's the difference between thinking and knowing. Once you know, it can't get better. I will do something for you though. Let's put them three shiny coins back in and see what comes out."

Again, the children's faces gave the answer. The white cloth swallowed the money and paid back three lollipops for the kids and another bag of bonbons.

"I thought I told you, 'Never give something back.' Do you ever listen?" That's when I noticed he'd done the trick over the lollipop jar. "Now girls, make sure he shares those. Bye for now, my beauties."

Once he came in with a bad chest and a rough mood. He gave me a tablet jar with a single penicillin capsule in it.

"Give us a few of those, would you? It's terrible that I am today. And tomorrow's a Tuesday. Please, young man, don't leave me bad on my Tuesdays. I'll pay all you want."

I half knew or had a sense that his doctor wouldn't mind, but I tried to persuade him all the same.

"Oh, now don't make me do that. I've only enough to pay yourself. And tomorrow's a Tuesday. Please, Jack, don't leave me bad on my Tuesdays. Oh, and listen, give me another one of those blue yolks. It's just that my chest is in bits. I left the last one down in Shannon."

I rang the doctor and again got the laughter. "Give them to him and whatever else he wants. Give that to him too. Sure, what's the point in me seeing him?

He'll just tell me what to write and how Tuesdays are his favourite day and all his money is spent on some boat in Shannon. Last time I got paid a duck egg. Tell him it was gone off."

The following month, late December, Helena had a brainwave. She took in his script and wrote "The Magic Man" in brackets beside his name and that's how it happened. Pat finally got entered in the computer. The bag label said, "Pat The Magic Man; address: Shannon."

I'd never seen the magician laugh before. Pat read the label over and over, each time taking small steps that stopped with a giggle and a half turn. He kept rearranging his hat, and then his half-smile finally opened and I saw joy. He called Helena and whispered in her ear. She blushed but nodded and went into the dispensary. At that moment, some traveller kids came in shouting. Normally, they'd break your heart, and that was putting it kindly, but for the following 10 minutes all was silent as Pat gave a magic show you could only dream of. To this day, that's the only time I've ever seen travellers stand still.

Helena and Trish came back from the dispensary, all smiles and with a bag for Pat. He wrote something on a piece of paper and gave it to Helena. She blushed again and showed it to Trish, who cracked up.

"My beauties, you've cheered me right up. Tomorrow's going to be a great Tuesday. You make sure that young fella looks after you! Helena, my dear, and Trish as always, it's my pleasure!"

Afterward, I found out that he just wanted more of those labels printed with his newly adopted surname. Helena gave him a whole label roll.

Pat became one of those people for whom you would bend or break or ignore just about every dispensing rule ever invented. And the best part was you never felt bad about it. ●

Tylenol Overdose

Mark Garofoli, PharmD, MBA

I had the following dialogue with a patient:

Patient: Doc, what do ya recommend for back pain?

Me: Well, have you tried anything already?

Patient: Yah, Tylenol, but it didn't work.

Me: How many did you "try"?

Patient: [pondering, and pondering more] I believe 56 yesterday.

Me: Fifty-six, 5, 6, right?

Patient: Yes, and about 20 or so today by around noon.

Me: How may I ask did you go about taking the 56 yesterday? Was it most at once, or building up?

Patient: Well, I took 3 or 4, and they didn't work, so I took 3 or 4 more 15 minutes later. Then when they didn't work, I took some more about a half an hour or an hour later, and so on, and so on.

Me: Well, I do have good and bad news for you. The good news is that as of right now you don't have to worry about your back pain, and rest assured, nothing is terribly wrong with you at the moment. The bad news is that you have overdosed on Tylenol and need to be seen by a hospital or clinic. I can call for transportation for you, or if you would like to arrange that for yourself via whatever means possible or necessary, that would be okay too. Again, there is no need to worry, as you can and will be taken care of after we take some measures to have you seen as soon as we possibly can.

Patient: Wow, this sounds pretty serious.

Me: Well, sir, yes, it is serious. Within 1 day, your skin may start turning yellow, and your body will actually start shutting down in another day. So, this is very serious. But, as I assured you, you can and will be taken care of and don't need to worry at all, really, as long as we follow up correctly. So, would you like me to call you a cab or an ambulance if you'd like?

The patient went to the local hospital. Two days later, he came back and gave me the greatest compliment a pharmacist could ever receive. He said, "Doc, I'm alive and I owe it to you!"

For pharmacists, the important questions are the ones that are not asked every time of every patient but should be (as in, Have you tried anything for that problem yet?). ●

The Journey Versus the Destination

Christa M. George, PharmD, BCPS, CDE

The first time I met Patient X, he was lying in a hospital bed, surrounded by a sea of white coats. He was tired, irritable, and in pain—understandable for someone who had just received a liver transplant. We were rounding in the early morning on New Year's Day, and I was lamenting the fact that I had to work on a holiday. Having started the job only 2 months before, the long, intense days had already worn me out. I was at the bottom of a steep learning curve and had little confidence that I would make it to the top. I was out of my element, practicing in an inpatient setting with no prior training in transplantation. In short, I had no idea what I was doing.

Despite my best efforts to the contrary, I found Patient X's irritability to be incredibly annoying. "Shouldn't this kid be grateful to be alive?" I thought. The team attributed his moodiness to the corticosteroids he was receiving and to his young age. I noticed that he was born the same year that *Star Wars* was released and suddenly realized how young he was. He reminded me of a younger cousin around the same age who was like a little brother to me. My mood softened, and I resolved to return the next day with a new attitude.

Over the next several days, we discussed his numerous medications, the indications, dosing, side effects, and drug interactions. Gradually, I came to know his parents, friends, and girlfriend. They were a close-knit, supportive group. We conversed easily as we planned for his discharge. His transplant was a success; everyone expected him to return to his "normal" life. We could not have anticipated what was ahead.

Nine months later, I began practicing in the outpatient transplant clinic. I had gained confidence in my knowledge and skills, and I was thrilled to be out of the hospital. Alongside a nurse practitioner, I assumed responsibility for the care of several hundred liver transplant patients. The days were long and ever changing; one day a patient could be stable and the next experience organ rejection. Because of the need for frequent follow-up, I would often speak to or see patients several times a week. Patient X was no different. I soon came to know his true personality: funny, friendly, happy to be alive. He began to tell me his story. He had graduated from college and wanted to find a good job and raise a family.

He played guitar occasionally. He and his girlfriend were getting serious and contemplating marriage. My nurse practitioner colleague and I began to refer to him as "our boy," treating him like the kid brother that neither of us had.

Several months later, I entered his hospital room while he was receiving treatment for a rejection episode. His girlfriend was sitting next to him on the bed while he had a Thymoglobulin infusion running into his arm. Despite frustration with being in the hospital, he was giddy with excitement. "We're getting married!" he exclaimed, smiling. The rejection had thwarted their plans to take a cruise, during which he had planned to propose. It was thrilling to see him happy and living his life to the fullest. I was truly disappointed when I could not attend the wedding because of a family commitment.

"It's all right. You were there in spirit," he said.

Time passed, and overall Patient X did well. He found a good job and settled into married life. Still, he grew frustrated at the occasional mood swings that were likely related to his continued need for prednisone. Because he had experienced a few episodes of mild rejection, the team felt that his risk for organ loss was too great to stop the drug. We adjusted his drug regimen and prescribed the lowest effective dose of prednisone.

The next year, when his son was born, I went to his parents' house to see the baby. The family was ecstatic. Everyone felt intense emotion that day, knowing how lucky he was to be able to look into the eyes of his son.

Three years later, the time came for me to move on. I wanted to return to outpatient internal medicine, where I could focus on my true therapeutic interest, diabetes. It had been a long 3 years, full of intense joy and loss. I had made lifelong friendships and learned a great deal about myself. I had gained confidence in my clinical skills and was beginning to learn to accept the things about patients that I could not control.

Of all my patients, it was Patient X that I dreaded telling the most. "It's all right. I'm happy for you," he said.

A year later, my former colleague called. "Patient X is in the clinic today. You should walk over and say hello." I walked into the room and looked into the smiling face of his son, who was now 2 years old.

Patient X introduced us by saying to his son, "This is Christa. She's one of the reasons Daddy's alive." I shrugged it off, but inside I was deeply moved. It was wonderful to see him so happy. It would turn out to be the last time I would see him.

Patient X and I kept in touch through phone and e-mail, although our conversations grew less frequent as time passed. I received occasional updates from my colleague: He had another mild rejection and was developing other complications. His mood swings had become more frequent, and he had begun seeing a psychiatrist. Eventually, he and his wife separated. I thought about contacting him but did not. I didn't know what to say. I couldn't fix this. I didn't have any answers for him. I asked my former colleague to tell him I asked about him.

Four years after the last time I saw him, my former colleague called. "It's our boy," she said, and I knew that he was gone. Ultimately, the inability to return to his previous "normal" life became too much for him. The fact that Patient X ended his life the same way that he lived it—on his own terms—offered no comfort. I thought of his son and hoped that the knowledge of how much his father loved him would one day fill the hole left by his father's absence.

I am thankful to have known Patient X, if only for a short time. He showed me that although our goal as pharmacists is to help patients achieve a positive outcome, the true joy of caring for others is found in the moments along the journey, whatever the outcome. ●

Patient-Centered Care: Changing Lives

Sarah T. Melton, PharmD, BCPP, CGP

I have the pleasure of working in an ambulatory care setting in a rural, medically underserved region. I am a psychiatric pharmacist and see patients with a variety of mental health and addiction issues. The wait to see a psychiatrist is often 4 to 6 months, and most patients present to their primary care providers for treatment while waiting for a psychiatry consult. I work with primary care physicians in a collaborative practice to provide needed psychiatric care as a "bridge" for patients in the months leading up to their psychiatry visit.

Pharmacists are trained medication experts, but adjusting medications will only get you so far in the realm of therapeutic outcomes. Developing skills in delivering care that is truly patient-centered is imperative for obtaining the best possible outcomes. Patient-centered care considers patients' cultural traditions, their personal preferences and values, their family situations, and their lifestyles.

I recently met two young patients whose treatment exemplifies these principles. If I simply met with the patients and their families and only looked at their medications, I am certain neither would have made the improvements that I have documented over the past year.

Susan came to me from a primary care physician in another town. Her mother could not wait 6 months for her to see a psychiatrist who would accept Medicaid payment. Susan is 22 years old and has mild mental retardation. She always has a shy smile on her face, but when she speaks, her voice booms loudly across the office. Susan graduated from high school at age 19, but she cannot read or write. Her medications were thrown haphazardly into a Mickey Mouse tote bag, and neither she nor her mother was able to tell me the names of the medications. However, she seemed to be taking most of her psychiatric medications on the appropriate schedule. Her medications for diabetes and blood pressure, though, were hit or miss.

Susan was diagnosed with attention deficit hyperactivity disorder (ADHD) at age 5 and had been on high doses of methylphenidate since then. She had never had a drug holiday. Over the years, more and more medicines were added on to combat adverse effects from the stimulants. These included a mood stabilizer for irritability, which caused her weight to skyrocket; a sedating antipsychotic to help her sleep, which contributed to weight gain and diabetes; and an ACE inhibitor for hypertension. Her behavior, diet, and sleep schedules had become out of control, and her mother was at the end of her rope.

Susan and I had something in common that made us bond from the first visit: we were "shoe-aholics." She loved my shoes, and I loved hers, and the topic of new shoes always starts our conversations. With every patient I meet, I try to find something that interests them to start the conversation. This approach helps the transition into discussing topics that are more difficult.

With Susan, we ordered all of her medications in blister packs to help with adherence and tapered off the high-dose methylphenidate over a month. We adjusted her diet and developed an incentive chart with stars for her mother to use for behavior and exercise. Within a couple of weeks off the stimulants, her blood pressure had improved, she was sleeping better, and the irritability was much improved. The exercise program and incentives for good behavior were also effective; she lost 3 pounds in the first 2 weeks and had enough stars to be able to purchase a new pair of shoes.

I think what bothered me most about this case was that Susan could not read or write. This situation significantly contributed to holding her back socially. I called our local literacy program and got Susan enrolled. She now attends the program 3 days a week for one-on-one assistance with reading and is making good progress. She is working at the local grocery store 2 afternoons a week. Clearly, a focus on only the methylphenidate would never have gotten Susan as far as she has come.

Another patient, Donnie, was referred to me for medication management when he was expelled from kindergarten in the last 2 weeks of the school year. He had been evaluated and diagnosed with ADHD in the past 3 months and was started on atomoxetine and clonidine. He had made no improvement since starting the medications and, in fact, had become more difficult to control. He hit his teacher at school, was not producing any satisfactory work, and cursed the principal with language that is difficult to hear an adult say, much less a small 5-year-old. When I first saw him, he rolled back and forth across the exam room on a stool, banging repetitively into the wall. My students looked at me with dismay and wondered how in the world we could ever help this child.

The mother looked exhausted as she bounced her 9-month-old boy on her lap who loved making the visit even more chaotic by letting out a high-pitched scream at regularly timed intervals. Clearly, more was going on in this family besides the fact that the medications were not working.

A full history revealed that the mother was recently remarried and there was great conflict with Donnie's father. Donnie was underweight and eating mainly processed foods and getting lots of caffeine, and he had no regular bedtime routine. He would not swallow any medications, and his mother was emptying atomoxetine capsules into pudding or applesauce to get him to swallow the medication. Some days he ate it, and some days he did not—no wonder no improvement had been seen.

The students and I completely changed his diet with his mother's cooperation. A strict bedtime routine was initiated. With regard to the medications, I had the atomoxetine and clonidine compounded into liquid form at a compounding pharmacy that had experience doing this for a child psychiatrist. I spent a great deal of time in educating the mother on how to administer the medication with the oral syringe, and Donnie did an excellent job in participating in this whole process. Within 2 weeks on the new regimen, Donnie was a new little boy. He was able to interact appropriately in the exam room, his aggressive behavior had ceased, and he was sleeping on a regular schedule. He proceeded to attend first grade and excel the entire year. In second grade, he made straight A's, and his mother called to let me know that he had placed second in the school spelling bee. He is currently being tapered off his medication to see whether he is able to sustain the progress made over the past 2 years.

When you make the patients and their families an integral part of the health care team, it empowers them to participate in making care decisions. When you provide them with the proper tools and support, patients are more likely to be adherent with their medications and treatment plan and to make healthful life decisions. As a pharmacist providing patient-centered care, the joy of seeing the quality of life of a patient dramatically improve is very rewarding. ●

Med Check

Robert A. Lytle, RPh

Years ago, an event occurred that springboarded me into a new career, or so I hoped at the time.

One of my elderly customers called and asked me to fill her prescriptions.

"All right," I said, "what are the numbers of the ones you need?" As I was saying this, I was pulling up her file on the computer.

"I can't really see the labels that well," she said, "just fill everything."

This type of request invariably results in anxious moments at the counter when the customer arrives and says, "Oh, I didn't need that one or that one or that one." Then, I have to undo all the ones the customer doesn't want.

So I said, "Let me go over the list."

Sure enough, when I got to her diabetes drug, she said, "No, I don't need that one."

I checked the date of its last fill. It had been 3 months. She really should have been out of it. "No," she said, "I've got plenty of those."

I guessed that maybe she had gotten samples from her doctor, so I dismissed that one and made notes to fill the rest. Then she added, "Oh, and could you please bring them out to me. I'm tired and not feeling very well today. I don't think I should drive."

I told her the medications would be delivered. That might have been the end of the story, except for one thing: I was not only her pharmacist, I was also her delivery boy.

That afternoon, I took her pills to her and she, as usual, invited me in. I was still wondering about her diabetes med, so I asked her about it.

"No, see?" she said, producing a bottle from her purse and shaking it to show me it was full.

I checked the label. It *was* for glyburide, all right, but it was from several years ago. I popped it open and found, I don't know, aspirins, saccharine pills, capsules—a hopeless variety of other things—including an occasional glyburide.

"I've been taking one twice a day like it says," she said triumphantly.

The pieces of the puzzle suddenly fell into place. Her poor vision, malaise, tiredness—all could be attributed to the lack of her proper dose of glyburide.

When I pointed out my discovery, she stared at me, as if suddenly remembering something. "Oh, Bob. Last year when I visited my sister, I lumped all of my pills into one bottle. I was only going to be gone for a week, and I didn't want to take so many bottles. I bet all of those pills are old."

"They're not just old," I said. "They're wrong."

I went back to the store and brought her a refill of the glyburide.

I wish *that* had been the end of the story, but it wasn't. She died a month later due to complications from her diabetes.

The incident prompted me to question the sufficiency of what most of us consider diligent efforts to provide our customers with proper health care. How many other situations like this would I find if I visited my customers' homes?

I was soon to find out.

Our community has a senior commission that oversees a variety of programs for the elderly. I called them and offered to make visits to those they felt might need some in-home medical supervision.

For the next several months, I made personal visits. Boy, were my eyes opened!

One man had told the agency that he had periodic bouts with poor health. When I got to his place, he had his entire assortment of pills on a lazy Susan in the center of his kitchen table—dumped in small open dishes. There was not a pill bottle in sight. "Oh, I can't get those danged tops off," he said, "so every couple months, a neighbor boy comes around and pops them open for me."

That visit happened to be in July. The temperature and humidity were both in the upper 90s. I cringed when I realized that his periodic bouts of ill health undoubtedly were due to the gradual impotence of his meds. I suggested he ask his pharmacist to provide easy-open tops with his next set of refills.

Another visit took me to the house of a man who revealed that he couldn't be bothered with taking his pills four times a day, so he took them all at once.

A woman said her heart was fine, so she only took her digoxins when she felt she needed them.

Another woman stored her pill bottles in the bathroom medicine cabinet. The labels were so wrinkled from humidity that they almost fell off the bottles, which, for the sake of convenience, were propped open on the shelf.

With almost every home visit, I made similar discoveries, and I realized that none of these life-endangering situations could have been revealed without a trained professional's personal home visit. "Brown-bag" programs are fine—they can expose obvious drug incompatibilities, but sometimes that's not enough. A regular home visit by someone who knows what to look for can make all the difference in a person's well-being.

This experience led to my "change in career" that I mentioned.

At the suggestion of an elderly friend and customer, I wrote a book that described the various pitfalls of managing medications. The deal was that I would visit peoples' homes, gather case studies, write the book, and get it published. My friend was a retired benefits manager and had all sorts of contacts in the business and insurance world. It would be his job to land contracts with those sources, and we would sell the book like crazy! We would both be millionaires in no time.

So I got busy, wrote the book, paid a bunch of money to get it published, and had it delivered—all 5,000 copies—to my store's basement. At exactly that point, my business partner had a heart attack and died. Since I had neither the ability nor the inclination to market my gold mine, I decided to cut my losses and stick with the day-to-day world of retail pharmacy.

I still have about 4,900 little blue books gathering dust with very little hope of ever seeing the inside of their intended market's homes.

If anyone out there needs some kindling, I know where you can find it. ●

The Things Patients Bring Us

Michelle Zingone, PharmD, BCPS

The pharmacist involved in anticoagulation management tends to have patients who are outwardly paranoid about bleeding. Because of this, they usually notify the pharmacist of the slightest bit of blood they see.

One day, a patient brought me a pink plastic cup that was sealed with plastic wrap and a rubber band. I saw the patient holding it in her hand, but she made no reference to its contents. I began my questioning with the typical items, confirming her current warfarin dose and asking about medication changes, vitamin K intake, acute illness, signs of thrombosis, and, finally, signs of hemorrhage. When I arrived at the final item, she handed me the pink plastic cup and instructed me to unwrap the plastic covering. I asked her to tell me what was inside, but she insisted that I open it first. I could tell from looking through the plastic wrap that it was not a solid object and, having a decent tolerance to bodily excretions, I felt I would be able to handle whatever it was.

When I unwrapped the cup, I found about 10 mL of sputum. I did not see any problem with the sample, so I questioned why she had brought it to me. She said she thought that there was "a lot of blood" in the sample. Because she collected the sputum in a pink plastic cup, the entire sample appeared pink as well. I could see no overt signs of blood in the sample, but the patient insisted that I take it to a physician to examine.

I brought the sputum sample to one of the physicians in the practice, and he immediately asked what I was doing and told me to throw the sample away. I told the physician that the patient was convinced she was going to die because of the "blood" in her sputum, and I asked him to reassure her that this was not the case.

When we arrived back in the exam room, the patient was shocked to see the physician and thought that meant he was the bearer of bad news. After he told her that the sputum sample was nothing to worry about, she had a look of relief on her face. We quickly concluded the visit and sent the patient on her way. ●

The Cost of Medications ... and Necessary Sacrifices

Heather Eppert, PharmD, BCPS

As a pharmacy intern functioning as a pharmacist in a small-town rural health clinic, I was often asked to find assistance for patients' medications through various outlets. One particular patient was well known to our clinic because he had been treated for heart disease, chronic obstructive pulmonary disease, and diabetes. One day, the physician informed me that it was time for the patient to get "serious" about taking his medications. The patient reported that he couldn't afford his medications and that the doctor would need to figure out a way to get the medications for him if he really expected him to take them. As usual, the doctor came to my office to ask for assistance. I confirmed with the doctor that several options were available for the patient and proceeded to spend hours completing the appropriate paperwork. Four weeks later, all the patient's medications arrived, ready for pickup at the clinic.

I contacted the patient every day for several weeks, with no success. I left message after message, but he never called back. I even sent the patient several letters by mail, asking him to come to the clinic to get his medications. I spoke with the patient's physician numerous times. The physician and I were exasperated but at the same time concerned that something may have happened to the patient.

Several weeks passed, and the patient was scheduled to be in the office the next day for a follow-up appointment with the physician. I reminded the physician that the medications were in the clinic, waiting for the patient, and that I desired to speak with the patient and provide his education on his new medications. The next day, the physician confronted the patient about the medications and asked why he had not returned the messages or letters that were sent to him. The physician asked the patient, "Why didn't you have the courtesy to call the pharmacy intern back?"

The patient replied, "Yeah, well, I suppose I should have. But you see, I didn't have money for gas, so I wouldn't have been able to come to pick up the medications anyway." The physician reinforced to the patient the importance of taking his medications and managing his chronic diseases. The patient told the physician, "Well, you see, it's all just too expensive, I can't afford it."

The physician replied, "Well, I've asked you to stop smoking, which would save you a lot of money, but you won't. I guess you're just going to have to stop eating—you need to lose weight anyway." The education and counseling session that followed was an interesting one, to say the least. ●

Stop Needling Me!

Donald Rolls, RPh

One of the areas that pharmacists must be vigilant about is drug and drug-device diversion—that is, obtaining a drug or drug device under false pretenses for illegal purposes.

One day while working at a popular retail chain pharmacy, a woman in her early 30s approached the pharmacy counter and asked to purchase a package of insulin syringes. Our store policy in the past was to sell this item without a prescription and without question. Our new policy, however, restricted the sale of all syringes to prescription only. When I told her of the new policy, she became very angry and immediately wanted to speak to the pharmacy supervisor. When I told her she was already speaking to him, she launched into an impassioned speech and accused me of preventing her from taking care of herself. "What kind of pharmacist would stand in the way of good patient care?" she screamed. "You're here to serve your patients!"

When I asked her what type of insulin she used and the dosage, her answer floored me. "I don't use insulin!" she protested, "I need these syringes for my crystal meth! I'm trying to prevent the spread of disease by using clean needles, and you're giving me a hard time!"

Well, how do you respond to that? I told her that although I appreciated her conscientiousness when it came to public safety, I wasn't there to enable her and other addicts to engage in a dangerous, destructive, and illegal practice. I offered to provide information on treatment programs as well as skin and oral hygiene advice for her increasingly deteriorating skin and teeth, but she wouldn't hear of it.

"I thought this pharmacy was supposed to care about us, but I see now that you don't. It's all about your stupid little laws!" she exclaimed. And with that, she threw the loaf of bread she was carrying at me and stormed out. I never saw her in the store after that. ●

The Phone

Pamela Stewart-Kuhn, RPh, MPA, CGP

I work in a small but busy military pharmacy. About half of our business is processing refill prescriptions. We have a phone-in refill system that consists of voice mail, where patients are instructed to leave their names and prescription numbers for us to fill. It's a common, yet less sophisticated system than that used by most military pharmacies. Most patients manage fine with leaving a simple message. However, some patients get flustered, can't hear on the phone, or just plain don't want to call an answering machine. Henry is one of those patients.

He called the pharmacy's main number to complain that the refill line wasn't working. I insisted that it was working, and we had been taking the refills off the recorder all day. He was so adamant that he was right that he came down to the pharmacy with the handset of his home phone with him. He handed me the handset and insisted that I call the refill line from his home phone. As he handed me the handset, it suddenly dawned on him that the base to the phone was 9 miles away at his home. There isn't a digital or analog phone anywhere that will connect to a base 9 miles away. I managed not to laugh at him (at least until he left) and processed his refill while he waited. •

The Pooh Room

Michelle Zingone, PharmD, BCPS

As a pharmacist now working in a physician's office, I see patients bring a variety of gifts to their physicians to show their appreciation for the services provided. These items range from freshly cut flowers to home-baked goods. Pharmacists are also recipients of such gifts, but recently, I have received other types of "gifts" from patients.

As relatively new additions to a private family medicine practice, two other pharmacists and I acquired space in a room that was originally decorated for pediatric patients. It contains a wallpaper border and a kite of Winnie the Pooh. Because of this, the room has been nicknamed the "Pooh Room."

We see an older couple on a regular basis for the wife's anticoagulation therapy. She is 78 years old with recent onset of dementia, which seems to worsen each time I see her. During one appointment with the couple, she said she had something to show me. I told her I would take a look at whatever it was once I got her settled in the exam room. She always carries a messenger bag (in place of a purse) because it's easier for her to carry with her four-wheeled walker. The item she wanted to show me, however, was not placed in her messenger bag. Instead, it was resting on the built-in seat of her walker.

When the patient and her husband were settled in the exam room, I asked what it was she wanted to show me. Her husband quickly stood up and said he would have to leave the room for this. I figured he was being respectful to his wife, and I did not think much of it. Once he left the room, she reached for a gallon-sized plastic bag on her walker. There was a neatly folded piece of fabric inside the bag, so I was not able to see what she was about to show me. When she opened the plastic bag, I needed no other sense but my sense of smell. She had brought me a sample of her stools!

She had been collecting her stools for the past few days because, as she stated, "It usually comes out in one piece, but now it's coming out in these small balls." The stool sample matched nicely to the Bristol Stool Scale type 1 (separate hard lumps, like nuts; hard to pass). She had managed to collect a day's worth of stools and wrap them neatly in the piece of fabric, which I recognized to be a pillowcase. I figured that she thought she had some gastrointestinal bleeding, because we talk about monitoring of stools at each visit. I finally realized she was trying to demonstrate to me that she was experiencing constipation.

The stench in the room was beginning to overwhelm me, so I told the patient that I needed to talk with her primary care physician. However, before I left, I knew I would somehow have to contain the smell (without offending the patient), so I kindly asked her to dispose of the stools in the biohazard waste bin (which luckily had a lid). When I said this, the patient began to drop the stools; they fell first on her lap, then on the chair, and eventually to the floor. I immediately gloved up and grabbed as many paper towels as possible and began picking them up. The patient, again with her worsening dementia, began to help me gather the stools with her bare hands. We eventually got all of the stools contained in the biohazard bin, and I left the exam room, asking the patient to wash her hands.

The patient's primary care physician has exam rooms on the other side of the office, well away from the radiating smell of the exam room the patient was in. I reported to her that the patient was experiencing constipation, and we agreed to have her start taking docusate sodium.

I then made my way back to the exam room. Her husband had rejoined us for the remainder of the visit. The next thing I needed to do was prick her finger for a blood sample for an international normalized ratio, or INR, test. I was not 100 percent sure that the patient had washed her hands in the time that I was out of the exam room, so I took it upon myself to wash both of her hands with isopropyl alcohol before I prepared my supplies for testing. The rest of the appointment was conducted without a hitch. The patient and her husband were told to return in 2 weeks for their follow-up visit.

When they left the office, the exam room still had an odor, and it would have been inappropriate to continue to use the room for patient care until it was taken care of. Because of this, I needed to empty the biohazard waste bin to remove the source of the odor, disinfect all the areas of the exam room the stools had touched, and disinfect the air in the room. The providers who had exam rooms next to this one were complaining of the odor radiating into their rooms, but there was no way for me to contain the smell. To my relief, the next scheduled patient hadn't arrived for the appointment, which provided me with ample time to clean, disinfect, and deodorize the room for the remaining patients of the day.

Now, when we make reference to seeing patients in the "Pooh Room," the nickname has a whole new meaning! ●

Quinidine: Left the Scene

Michael J. Schuh, PharmD, MBA

I had a very impatient regular customer urging me to hurry up with his prescription. This was not new for him, but he was more impatient than normal that day. I could never understand why someone who lived literally behind the store and who was retired and in the store virtually every day could always be in such a hurry to get his refills.

I was just finishing the prescription when suddenly, without a word, the man turned and walked away up the aisle in front of my position in the pharmacy. From the look of the rear of his white shorts, I could see he had an accident. Looking down again to the prescription, I saw it was for quinidine sulfate. Now I understood why he was always so impatient. He suffered from abrupt diarrhea, a well-known side effect of quinidine.

Although I never saw him again, I know that sometimes people ask more of us because of necessity. ●

Shorted in Spring Hill

Michael J. Schuh, PharmD, MBA

When much younger and freshly out of school and trying to buy our first house, I worked many, many days in a row for my employer to save enough money for my wife and I to buy that house. So, I worked on my days off at many of my chain employer's stores all up and down the west coast of Florida.

I was working in Spring Hill one day and got an irate phone call from a woman who said she was shorted one hydroxyzine tablet on her prescription. Being the good chain pharmacist I was, I placed the woman on hold and told the technician to type (yes, type) another label and to place another tablet in a bottle so she could come and get it at no charge, thinking we had accidently miscounted her prescription.

I was informed by the technician that this woman did this on *every* prescription she got, no matter who the pharmacist was, and that she was continually getting free medications. It had been long established in the pharmacy that everyone double count all her medications to be sure she was not shorted, but she always called shortly after she left to say she had been shorted. The technician added that the woman waits for other patrons to be around the cash register and then rushes up with her loud and theatrical complaint on how the pharmacy staff was always cheating her out of her medicines.

After hearing this information, I had an idea. I got back on the phone with the woman and told her that we absolutely did not miscount or short her any medicine and that I would count the tablets right in front of her. "We'll see about that!" she shouted on the telephone. I was met with a blank stare by the technician before she asked what I was going to do, knowing the woman would have removed the one tablet before she got to the store.

Fifteen minutes later, as the usual crowd of patrons gathered around the register at 5 pm to pick up their prescriptions, she appeared. We didn't notice her at first because of the crowd and she was off to the side waiting for the right moment to perform. I didn't know which person she was, but the technician nudged me as soon as she spotted this well-known patron.

When the crowd was at critical mass, she loudly proclaimed our crime as she waded through the masses to get to the cash register, demanding to see the pharmacist who cheated her out of her pill.

I walked down to the checkout counter, counting tray and spatula in hand, and asked her for the bottle containing her hydroxyzine. "Don't you take the bottle back behind the counter," she exclaimed. "I want to see you count them right here!" So with Ms. Pugnacious Theatricalis and audience all around, I dumped her tablets onto the counting tray and slowly counted by fives to 30 tablets exactly. "What! I know I … Let me see that!" she bellowed, as she grabbed the spatula out of my hand. She then counted the tablets four times to verify the count. She was dumbfounded. How can this happen?

Unknown to her and my technician, I decided to try a little sleight of hand using the small tablet size of hydroxyzine as my ally. Before carrying the counting tray and spatula down to the counter, I placed a hydroxyzine tablet in the joint skin fold between my right ring finger and palm. When I dumped the tablets on the counting tray at the register, I merely opened my hand when doing so to let the extra tablet naturally drop with the other 29 tablets from the bottle onto the counting tray.

Before Ms. Theatricalis sheepishly left—without apology I might add—I apologized to her for any misunderstanding.

I worked in this store again 6 months later and asked about our hydroxyzine lady. I was told she never accused the pharmacy of shorting her again. ●

The Ultimate Cheapskate

Pamela Stewart-Kuhn, RPh, MPA, CGP

I work at a small military pharmacy. Like many base pharmacists, I offer over-the-counter medications for patients with a physician's prescription. It has been our philosophy that some of these medications will ultimately save us some money if they are used in place of more expensive prescription alternatives. Most of the time, this has worked out well. However, a few thrifty patients (almost always retired) have no qualms about asking their physicians for prescriptions for just about anything.

The prescriptions for calcium and multivitamins don't bother me much, because most elderly patients I encounter don't have very good eating habits. I fill the occasional cough and cold products because they rarely require refills. However, I had to politely explain to the couple requesting a 3-month supply of throat lozenges that I didn't think 3 months' worth was necessary, but I would provide a few boxes to each of them with refills, just in case. (I don't have a problem telling my patients no sometimes, but I am polite about it.)

My favorite, unbelievable, over-the-counter request came from a man named Jim. He had brought in several over-the-counter prescriptions in the past, so I already knew he was thrifty. However, I was speechless when he presented me a prescription for a box of condoms, with refills. Now, I remember from my days as an intern in a veterans' hospital that some elderly men use condoms as a sort of backup plan for minor urinary incontinence. Jim wasn't elderly, though, and I had never filled any prescriptions for him for urinary retention medications. I figured they had to be for "recreational purposes." I did fill the prescription, in the interest of wellness and public health. I couldn't help but wonder, if a man was too cheap to buy his own condoms, then he wasn't likely to buy his date a nice dinner or flowers. ●

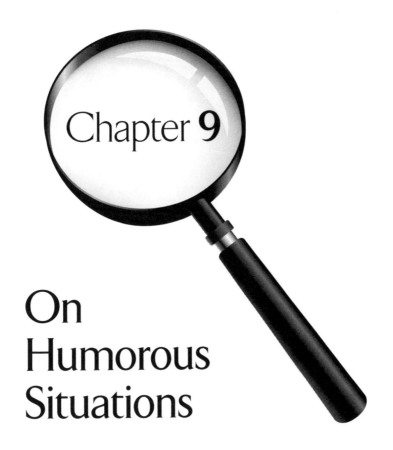

Chapter 9

On Humorous Situations

Always laugh when you can; it is a cheap medicine.

—Lord Byron

The Fine Art of Selling Condoms

J. Aubrey Waddell, PharmD, FAPhA, BCOP

I was 17 and a proud rising high school senior in the summer of 1975 when I was hired as a pharmacy technician, delivery boy, salesclerk, janitor, and what have you at North Hills Pharmacy, where my parents purchased their prescriptions. The pharmacy was located just outside of North Little Rock, Arkansas.

On Saturday afternoons, prescriptions were few and the business of the pharmacy was dominated by the selling of the wide variety of goods that the pharmacist-proprietor kept on hand. Commenting on his propensity to stock just about everything that the residents of the town might possibly need or want, a recent pharmacy graduate who was interning at the store said to me one day, "He keeps *way* too much junk in this place!"

One of the things my boss liked to provide for the neighborhood (seems so ironic now) was a fairly large selection of cigars, which I now realize were all cheap American cigar brands. I don't know the manufacturer of the cigars that are the complicating factor of this story, but these particular cigars were called "Trojans" and they lived with all the other cigars in the glass case that doubled as the front counter of the store.

On this particular Saturday afternoon, I was stationed at the cash register at that front counter. A tall young man entered the store, quickly caught my eye, and, in a confident and businesslike voice, said, "Hi there, I need a box of Trojans."

Now, it must be mentioned here that I had a very strict Missionary Baptist upbringing. Concerning the list of subjects that my parents Ed and Hazel Waddell decided I needed no formal training on was the various brands of condoms. Therefore, the only Trojans I knew, other than the famous ones from ancient Troy or the mascots of the University of Southern California or the University of Arkansas at Little Rock, were the Trojan cigars in that glass case. I quickly whipped a box of them out, placed them on the counter, and said, "That'll be X dollars" (obviously, I have long forgotten the price).

The man stared at me for a couple of seconds and then burst out laughing. He said, "Man, that is *hilarious*!" When he calmed down from laughing, he said, "Really, though, I'm in a hurry, and I need a box of Trojans."

I proceeded to the little office in the back corner of the pharmacy, where I knew my boss was counting money and reconciling charge accounts. Standing in the door, I asked sheepishly, "Other than a cigar, what have we got in here that would be called a Trojan?" Up to this point, my naiveté had been a source of fascination for him, but his expression told me that this was a new level of fascination in a man who was not easily fascinated.

He looked over his glasses at me and said, in a starkly verbless manner, "Condoms?" I shifted from foot to foot, oblivious to the meaning of that word. He tried again, "Rubbers?"

"Oh!" I said, "I know what those are! Really!" Then, I softened my voice, leaned toward him, and, almost in a whisper, said, "Where do we keep those?"

"In the last drawer to the right behind the prescription counter," he said.

"Why?" I asked.

He replied, "Because we are close to the high school. The high schoolers have a high demand for these things but don't want to be seen buying them, so they will steal them if I put them on a rack in the store."

Certain that I was now qualified as a man of the world, I went to the last drawer on the right behind the prescription counter. Eager with anticipation for this rite of passage, I opened the drawer and discovered another problem. The Trojan condoms came in a red box marked "regular" and a Carolina blue box marked "lubricated." Having no idea which type the man wanted, I leaned over the prescription counter and yelled across the crowded store, "Hey, you at the front, do you want *regular* or *lubricated*?" The man promptly left and, as far as I know, never did his condom business with North Hills Pharmacy again.

My boss walked up from behind, put his arm over my shoulder, and said, "Well, boy, I think it's time we had the talk about how to sell condoms."

Amazingly, the whole rest of the time I worked there, no one ever asked me for any condoms. Perhaps my reputation as a condom merchant became well known. Even though in 1975 we had not yet invented the phrase, I'm fairly certain that my unique set of condom-marketing skills had ended that pharmacy's contribution to the world of "safe sex." ●

ED Before It Was Called ED:
True Confessions of a Pharmacy Intern

W. Mike Heath, RPh, MBA

In the mid-1970s, I was a young pharmacist recently graduated from pharmacy school and had yet to start my career in the Army. I was working to complete my required internship hours at a community pharmacy, City Drug, in a small South Carolina town. The pharmacy, with its soda fountain and morning coffee ritual, was in many ways the focal point of the town, visited by numerous locals—predominantly men—who came to discuss the world's problems and render their opinions.

City Drug provided pharmacy services to a diverse population, many of whom were indigent and often obtained their chronic maintenance medications with whatever amount of money they could afford at the time. City Drug gave me numerous opportunities to interact with patients and improve my patient-communication skills.

One morning, an elderly patient arrived at the pharmacy, and I went to the over-the-counter section where he was waiting. "Sir, may I help you?" I asked politely.

He replied, "Yes, you can. My mule won't spit." His response caught me off guard, and although my grandfather was originally a farmer and I knew a little bit about animals, I didn't know a mule could spit.

Trying to be helpful, I asked, "Have you thought about taking your mule to a veterinarian?"

He looked at me, grinned with his head slightly bowed, and said, "No, not a real mule. My mule—I can't get it up." He went on to ask, "Don't you sell courage pills to help a man get it up?" Then, it dawned on me what he was talking about. City Drug did, in fact, sell vitamin B-1 (thiamine) tablets that for whatever reason had received the anecdotally based endorsement of helping a man "get it up," or, as we now know it, treat his erectile dysfunction, or ED.

I proceeded to meet the patient's needs, and as per City Drug protocol, I packaged and labeled a small bottle of vitamin B-1 tablets with the directions "Take as needed for courage." ●

A Tale from the Trenches

Charles D. Ponte, PharmD, CDE, BCPS, BC-ADM, FASHP, FCCP, FAPhA

If you want to be an effective educator, learn to be flexible and adapt to changing situations in the classroom or, for that matter, at the patient's bedside. Let me share with you a quick "tale from the trenches."

One afternoon, I was making pharmacy rounds on a hospitalized family medicine patient with two third-year baccalaureate pharmacy students assigned to my clinical rotation. I already had an established professional relationship with the patient, so I proceeded to sit next to him as he was lying in bed. I have found over the years that this "up close and personal" philosophy breaks down barriers, facilitates communication, and enhances rapport between the patient and the provider. I talked to the patient about how he was doing and some medication issues.

When I eventually got up to leave, I felt that my backside was wet. In truth, my white coat and pants were soaked. My light brown khaki pants had turned a dark brown. I must admit that I was somewhat embarrassed. I thought to myself, "I'm not incontinent, and my prostate is in good working order." Well, unknown to me at the time, the patient had urinated in bed and I had sat in the urine. Of course, my students thought that it was hysterical.

The moral of the story is "Watch where you sit," but it's also "Go with the flow," no pun intended. Laugh in the face of adversity. My students did! Of course, they had to repeat the rotation (just kidding). ●

Restaurant Chain Branching into Over-the-Counter Medications?

J. Aubrey Waddell, PharmD, FAPhA, BCOP

While in my oncology pharmacy residency at Walter Reed Army Medical Center in 1995–1996, I worked with an oncology fellow whose handwriting consisted of big, square letters. This was a good thing, because it made her medication orders easy to read. One day, an oncology pharmacy technician approached me with an order from this physician. He said, "Have you ever heard of Hooters Tylenol-containing products?" I told him I most certainly had not and asked him why he wanted to know. He handed me the physician's order, and the first line clearly read "No Hooters Tylenol-Containing Products."

Thinking this might be a perception problem on the part of the technician or myself, I showed the order to two other pharmacists, four nurses, two other pharmacy technicians, and three physicians, all of whom agreed that for some reason this patient was not to have any Hooters Tylenol-containing products. I was at a complete loss.

I finally approached the physician and asked her what she meant by her order. She grabbed the order from me, looked at it intently, and exclaimed, "That's not funny at all. This clearly says 'No Other Tylenol-Containing Products.' This patient has liver dysfunction!" Then, she turned and stomped away.

We made sure that the patient did not receive any products that contained acetaminophen. I still have a copy of that order in my files, and I take it out every so often to show students. For the life of me, it still says "No Hooters Tylenol-Containing Products." ●

Meeting a Louse with Poise and Professionalism

Nancy A. Alvarez, PharmD, BCPS, FAPhA

"I need a pharmacist at the window, please!" Once across the pharmacy threshold, I habitually answered to the name "pharmacist" instead of my own. So, upon hearing my "name," I began to make my way toward the "in" window. I worked for a major pharmacy chain, situated in a strip mall west of Phoenix, Arizona—before the craze of building large freestanding pharmacies on prime corner lots took over in 1994 or so. My pharmacy had long, narrow aisles, with just enough space for all the requisite equipment behind the counter, and it was a pretty tight fit for the staff of six on duty that day.

I arrived at the window to find a woman reaching into her purse. She removed a baby food jar sealed with plastic wrap. She set it down gently and with her index finger slid it across the counter. I bent down to meet the jar as it traveled toward me, finding myself eye to eye with a greenish-brown bug. "Are you kidding me?" I thought.

Before I could say anything, the woman asked, "Can you identify this for me? Can you tell what this is?"

I was waiting for someone to enter the window space and tell me this was a joke. I could see staff members migrating toward the computer terminals near the in window. I heard a snicker and a chuckle, and I wanted to giggle too. In fact, I was giggling on the inside. My preceptors had promised that I would have wacky practice experiences, but until this moment I did not believe them.

The woman then stated that she had found this bug on her child's head. Even though I did not know for sure, never having had an interest in entomology, I was fairly certain I was in the company of a louse.

Although I was amused to finally have a "crazy practice story" to share at cocktail parties, I waved off my staff with my hand, indicating for them to stop giggling and get back to their assigned stations to work. This was a pharmacy, and we were in the business of helping patients. I was cognizant that they were watching, and I wanted to reinforce the professional nature of our practice and to demonstrate that all requests were important, no matter how odd they seemed. This lady knew enough to ask her local pharmacist for assistance, and today that was me.

The various over-the-counter products used to treat head lice infestations were in sight over the lady's shoulder. I slid the baby food jar back across the counter and asked the woman to retrieve a product and return so that we could have a discussion. I listened to her concerns, answered her questions, and provided her with information on how to use the product and care for her home.

I was happy to be in a position to offer assistance to this woman and felt great satisfaction after our discussion. She thanked me and simultaneously slid the baby jar toward me again. "Can you do something with this back there?" One technician was swabbing down the counters with isopropyl alcohol and abruptly looked up, grinning ear to ear. Once again, I thought, "Are you kidding me?"

I smiled at the lady and calmly replied, "If you take this right outside of the store and let it out of the jar, it will likely be better served."

"Yes, you are probably right," she agreed, as she picked up the jar, placed it into her purse, and left the window.

This woman needed me to be the best professional I could be—as did my staff. Looking back, I believe that I was just that. ●

Donnatal on the Counter

Michael J. Schuh, PharmD, MBA

During my internship at a busy chain pharmacy, I observed gallon jugs of Donnatal Elixir under the prescription counter and asked my preceptor why we carried this medication in these quantities. He replied that it was a fast mover in the store, so they kept it in large amounts on the floor in that convenient location because the jugs were too heavy to keep on the shelf.

On one particularly busy day at the beginning of the month, I had to fill a Donnatal Elixir prescription. I reached down, picked up the nearly full gallon jug, and tapped it every so lightly on the edge of the counter. Boom! The jug exploded, sending bright green Donnatal all over the counter, prescriptions, pharmacy floor, and me. After a good laugh by all at my misfortune and after cleaning up the mess as best I could, I noticed a nice green hue to the floor and the entire, previously white, prescription counter. After the elixir dried, I found I could also stand my trousers up by themselves that night when I got home.

Three years later, when I returned to the same pharmacy as a pharmacist, the counter and floor were still a nice green hue. ●

Apply Locally

J. Aubrey Waddell, PharmD, FAPhA, BCOP

In the early 1990s, I was a captain in the U.S. Army Medical Service Corps and director of the pharmacy department of a military hospital in New Jersey. We had a busy outpatient pharmacy operation, averaging about 700 prescriptions per day. The operation had an "in" window staffed by a Red Cross volunteer, an order-entry computer workstation staffed by a technician, a filling line staffed by two technicians and a pharmacist, and an "out" window staffed by a pharmacist. Because my annual rating largely hinged on how satisfied our patients were with the outpatient pharmacy service, I spent a lot of time as the pharmacist at the out window, working hard to "quarterback" the operation and keep it as fast, accurate, and patient-friendly as possible. As hectic as the pace of work was, I did my best to answer medication questions from any patient who had them.

One day, a completed prescription for a topical cream was passed to me at the dispensing window. The directions on the label were "Apply locally twice a day," which matched the physician's order on the paper prescription. I called out the patient's name and a middle-aged man walked up to the window. After I checked his military identification as required, I handed him the medication and asked whether he had any questions about it. He replied that he did not, that this was a cream for his periodic outbreaks of poison ivy, and that he had used it before. He took the medication, thanked me, and read the label as he walked away. He stopped before he got to the door, read the label again, and walked back to me. He said, "It looks like the doctor wants me to apply this stuff locally. My wife and I wanted to go to the Pennsylvania Amish country tomorrow. Is that still considered local?" I honestly thought the man was joking, so I asked him how far into the Amish country he usually went and he replied that he and his wife usually stopped at Lancaster. I told him as long as he did not go past Lancaster, then it was still considered local. He thanked me again and walked away.

As the man departed, the other pharmacist said, "Captain, I think that man was serious." Alarmed, I ran out and caught him in the parking lot, and we shared a laugh at our mutual misunderstanding. After I thought about it, I realized that "apply locally" must seem to be a strange phrase to someone outside the medical field! •

Old Man Sneaking a Peek

Michael J. Schuh, PharmD, MBA

On weekends, when physician offices are closed, pharmacists are often required to triage patients for health problems. Should you recommend an over-the-counter product, have the patient see his or her doctor on Monday, or send the patient to the emergency room?

Late one Sunday afternoon while working alone in the pharmacy and answering a phone call, I noticed a woman in her mid-30s frantically waving at me from the cash register area. After hanging up, I walked down to the register to see what she needed. Before I could open my mouth, she yanked down her shorts and asked, "What's this?"

The store was empty of patrons except for this woman and an elderly man. He had noticed the waving, and subsequent exposure, at the register, so I asked the woman to step around the corner for more privacy. She had what looked like a large, port-wine birthmark lesion that apparently had cropped up suddenly. Thinking it could be an aggressive staphylococcus infection of some type, I explained that she should see a physician right away to get a diagnosis and treatment.

While discussing the lesion, we were both startled by a large crash behind us. It was Mr. Curiosity knocking over a floor display while trying to get a better look at the unfortunate, and partially clad, woman. ●

The Color of Poop

Pamela Stewart-Kuhn, RPh, MPA, CGP

I have a philosophy that I've developed over the years concerning my elderly patients. There comes a time in everyone's life when the production of a daily bowel movement, and the contents of that bowel movement, become an all-consuming issue. The age of onset does vary from person to person, with some starting in their 50s and others waiting until their 70s. Nonetheless, it seems to happen to everyone eventually.

I think one of the more interesting matters, from a pharmacist's perspective, is how closely this daily event is monitored. As a student, I read in the literature about certain dosage forms that would release medication into the gut, but the matrix would remain behind in the feces. I never gave it much thought. I can now report, with utter certainty, that patients do find pills, which are often brightly colored, in their poop. How do I know this? They feel compelled to bring the "recycled" pills into the pharmacy to prove it! ●

One Pitfall of Low-Cost Home Delivery

J. Aubrey Waddell, PharmD, FAPhA, BCOP

The smallest post I ever served on as a U.S. Army pharmacy officer was Yuma Proving Ground, Arizona. Although the actual land area of the proving ground was large, the part where people lived was very small. In fact, one trip around the post, using every street once, was a total of 5 miles. Because one of my hobbies is distance running, I found myself running this route a few times each week, when I wasn't doing longer runs along the many available desert roads.

Between the active-duty soldiers and family members on the post and military retirees from a nearby RV park, I filled 60 to 100 prescriptions a day at the pharmacy. At the end of the workday, I would sometimes have a few unclaimed prescriptions from residents of the post, because most of them worked during the day.

One day, an amazing idea hit me. Why not carry these prescriptions on a run, delivering them to their owners along the way? From then on, if I had unclaimed prescriptions, I placed them in small paper bags with the names and addresses of the patients written on the bags. Then, I changed into my running gear and ran the 5 miles, stopping a few times to knock on doors and deliver prescriptions to my patients. Not only did they appreciate it, but they also got huge laughs out of it, and I became somewhat of a local legend. No system is perfect, however, as I was to discover.

One morning, a young female patient well known to me came storming up to my pharmacy window and demanded to know who the young man was who ran by her house, stopped, walked up to her in her yard, handed her a bag containing her birth control pills, said goodbye, and ran away down her street the evening before? How did he get her prescription? Was it a habit of mine to give her prescriptions, which she correctly considered her private business, to complete strangers and tell them to take them to her house? And why did she want such strangers knowing where she lived in the first place? I'm telling you, this lady, who had always been very friendly and respectful to me, was tearing me to pieces, and I couldn't get a word in edgewise!

Finally, when she stopped for breath, I interjected, "Mrs. D, that was *me* who walked up and handed you your prescription in your yard last night."

She stared at me for a long time and then burst out laughing. "Well!" she exclaimed, "You certainly look different when you're running than when you're working here!"

For the rest of the time I was assigned at Yuma Proving Ground, I handed Mrs. D many of her prescriptions in her front yard. Every time, she laughed about the first time I provided her with such an unusual service. ●

Pride and Joy

Pamela Stewart-Kuhn, RPh, MPA, CGP

When I was a new pharmacist, just recently out of school, I learned early that it takes all kinds of people to make the world go around. At my retail pharmacy, it wasn't unusual to get to know some of the regular customers and hear about their spouses and children. One afternoon, an old man caught me off guard. He came into the pharmacy to pick up his medication. While I was ringing up his purchase, he asked me if I wanted to see his "pride and joy." I always tried to be courteous and figured he wanted to show me a picture of his wife, kids, or grandkids. He opened his wallet and showed me a photo—a box of Pride detergent set next to a bottle of Joy dish soap. He thought it was hysterical. I thought he had a rather twisted sense of humor. Needless to say, I passed on his offer the next time around! ●

The Soft Drink Machine

J. Aubrey Waddell, PharmD, FAPhA, BCOP

In the summer of 1975, when I was 17 and had just finished my junior year of high school, I was hired as a pharmacy technician, delivery boy, salescclerk, janitor, and what have you at North Hills Pharmacy, where my parents purchased our family's prescriptions. The pharmacy was located near our home in the unincorporated community of Sylvan Hills, which is now incorporated into the city of Sherwood, Arkansas.

One of my many duties was the nightly restocking of the pharmacy's soft drink machine. The machine was located in the middle of the store down the left-hand wall if one was facing the prescription counter in the back of the store. I took great pride in this duty. Stocking a soft drink machine seemed like such an adult endeavor to me, something I was proud to have people see me doing, especially young people. The more times I stocked the machine, the better I got to know the machine and all its functions and quirks. By August, I was the recognized expert on all matters related to the soft drink machine, and I reveled in this acknowledgment.

For example, whenever a customer put money in the machine and pressed one of the big rectangular buttons but did not receive one of the cold glass-bottled drinks, I was always summoned to diagnose and treat the problem. Most of the time, the treatment encounter went like this:

Me: So, when you pressed the button, did you hear a single sound like glass on metal, but then no more sound at all?

Customer: Yes.

Me: Well, you see, sometimes when the machine is full and you make a selection, the bottom bottle in the stack inside the machine falls a little too quickly and becomes wedged in the little opening it's supposed to fall through to make it to the door down here where you lift it out. Don't worry. I'll have it out in no time.

At this point, I would get down on my knees, open the little plastic door the bottles fell through under normal conditions, reach up into the machine, feel for and find the wedged bottle, and give the bottle a little flick with my extended fingers, causing it to fall neatly out the door. The customer would get the drink and walk away duly impressed at the expertise possessed by the staff of this fine pharmacy. Certainly, I reasoned, my service was building repeat business.

One hot August evening, I heard the familiar voice of the pharmacist-proprietor calling me to go to the soft drink machine, where a customer had just failed to complete a transaction. After a version of the conversation detailed previously, I got down on my knees and reached through the little plastic door up into the machine, located the stuck bottle, and gave it a little push with my fingers. However, an unexpected event occurred. As the bottle fell from its position, the other 20 bottles on top of it in the stack fell to the position vacated by the bottom bottle, and firmly and painfully wedged three of my fingers against the metal frame of the bottle stacker. The pain shot through my fingers and up my arm, and I started screaming in pain, struggling vainly to free my fingers. The stunned customer yelled, "He's being electrocuted by the machine!" and other customers gathered to watch the carnage, all of them apparently clueless on how to help me.

My boss dashed up the aisle and unplugged the machine, but I did not cease my screaming. He then realized that I was not being electrically charged, but was painfully stuck, and he ran to retrieve the keys to the machine. He opened it up and shouted to me, "What kind of drink was it?"

I shouted back, "Sprite!" He pulled out the 20 Sprites one by one as fast as he could, and my fingers were finally freed, although somewhat dented.

My boss retired some years later, and the store was never the same without him. It closed and was torn down shortly afterward, giving way to a new building for a church that had long shared the same property. To this day, though, every time I am home to visit my parents and I drive past that church, my fingers still hurt a little. •

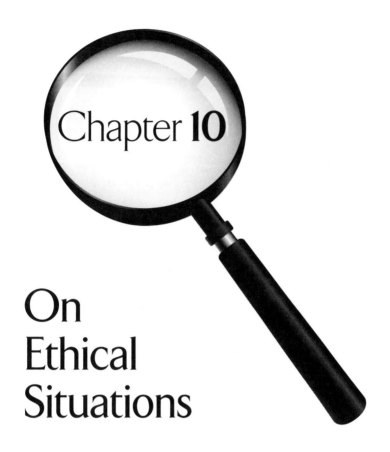

Chapter 10

On Ethical Situations

A pharmacist respects the autonomy and dignity of each patient.

> —From the Code of Ethics for Pharmacists,
> American Pharmacists Association

The Schindler of Pharmacy

Luigi Barlassina, MPharm Chemistry

His story is not as well known as that of Oscar Schindler, but like him, Tadeusz Pankiewicz is a hero—but a pharmacist hero.

When, under the German occupation of Poland during World War II, the Nazis established the Krakow Ghetto, Pankiewicz's pharmacy became the only such establishment within its boundaries. The Nazis offered Pankiewicz one of the Jewish pharmacies in Krakow, but he refused. He eventually was allowed to continue to run his pharmacy and take up permanent residence in the ghetto, becoming the only non-Jewish Pole living within the walls. His staff—Irena Drozdzikowska, Helena Krywaniuk, and Aurelia Danek—were given permits to enter and exit the ghetto for work.

Pankiewicz soon won acceptance and respect among the inhabitants of the ghetto. Open 24 hours a day, the Under the Eagle Pharmacy became a center of resistance to Nazi policy. It provided medical help, became a trusted location to host meetings and exchange information, and was a place to hide.

The scarce medications and pharmaceutical products supplied to the ghetto's residents were usually free of charge and substantially improved quality of life. More important, apart from health care considerations, the pharmacy staff contributed to survival itself. As Pankiewicz mentions in his memoir, he and his staff came up with some "tricks" that were able to help many people avoid deportation: they provided tranquilizers for children who were being hidden from the German soldiers during SS raids and hair dye for older people. Giving the elderly a more youthful look enabled them to avoid deportation to the death camps.

In the last tragic days of the ghetto, Pankiewicz and his staff were on hand to distribute medicines and dressings to residents. Everyone who turned to them for help received it.

Every day, Pankiewicz and his staff risked their lives to undertake numerous clandestine operations: smuggling food and information and offering shelter on the premises for Jews facing deportation to the camps.

Originally published in the *Irish Pharmacist*. Adapted with permission from GreenCross Publishing.

When the war ended, Pankiewicz continued to work at the pharmacy until 1953. He died on November 5, 1993, after being honored (as had Schindler) by the Israeli Holocaust Memorial authority Yad Vashem as one of the "Righteous Among the Nations."

Today, save for one stretch of wooden stalls, the original character of the pharmacy has been lost. It was closed in 1967, and its interior was altered when the building was converted into a restaurant. In 1983, the pharmacy became a branch of the Krakow Historical Museum, holding a permanent exhibition dedicated to showing the annihilation of Krakow's Jews by the Nazis and the role that Pankiewicz's pharmacy had in the ghetto. ●

Bibliography

Crowe DM. *The Holocaust: Roots, History, and Aftermath.* Boulder, CO: Westview Press; 2008.

Crowe DM. *Oskar Schindler: The Untold Account of His Life, Wartime Activities, and the True Story Behind The List.* New York, NY: Basic Books; 2007.

Martin G. *The Holocaust: A History of the Jews of Europe During the Second World War.* New York: Holt Paperbacks; 1987.

Pankiewicz T. *The Cracow Ghetto Pharmacy* (translation by Henry Tilles). New York: Holocaust Library; 1987.

Are You Sure?

Julian Judge, MPSI, BSc(Pharm), Dip Grad Psych

Jack had a number of issues here, and he knew it. The first was that Rachael had told him she had just turned 17, but he didn't believe her. She looked too young. The second was her positive result. He asked her to produce another sample to repeat the test. He told her it was just to check the first. The reality was it gave him time to think. It was still positive, as he knew it would be. A single straight line and as pink as pink could be.

He had a direct clash between her welfare and her need for confidentiality. She was adamant that nobody, especially her parents, be told. Yet, she had been in the back all afternoon and evening, nearly 6 hours. Initially, it was to calm her down, but as her distress got worse, it was more to calm Jack and the staff down.

It was now closing time. She was still crying and didn't want to leave.

Her cries had been loud and wretched at first but were now just quiet sobs. Earlier, eye shadow and lipstick streaked her face and hands. The girls cleaned it up. Her older friend had left, and she had to go to work. Jack had never seen tears like these before. No amount of assurance that all would be okay or hugs from the girls were helping. Simply put, at that moment, she wanted to stay in the dispensary forever.

Patient confidentiality was one thing, but Jack and the staff were resolute: She was in no state to be left alone. He swore to himself and vowed never, ever to offer a pregnancy testing service again. The year was 1992, and he was charging 3 pounds a test. The tests came in boxes of 50 and cost 50 pence each. At first, his only concern was their reliability. The rep gave him a full box of free samples.

Everybody tested themselves and each other. He knew one of his staff was pregnant. After a week of testing, she was still pregnant. The rest weren't, and neither was he. The rep was right: The tests were reliable. That was 2 months ago. Financially, it was worth it.

"Look Jack, everybody's going to win here. You'll provide a service that's needed and get a good margin. The test is 100 percent reliable. Your patients will get a quick result without having to go to the doctor, where it costs more. And

Originally published in the *Irish Pharmacist*. Adapted with permission from GreenCross Publishing.

if the result is positive, you can refer them to their doctors. So, the doctors get business too and they're happy. This is a good deal Jack," said the rep.

At the time, it seemed like a good idea. However, unforeseen problems emerged. The main one being that Jack was young and naive. Another was that he had just opened his pharmacy, was under financial pressure, and had not thought things through.

Politically speaking, the local doctors weren't too happy about it, especially the closest one. They weren't mad, but they weren't jumping for joy either. "This is a community and not a high street," one doctor, whom Jack liked, had said. "Look Jack, your prices are going to be a lot cheaper than mine, and that's fine. Just be sure you know what you're letting yourself in for here. It's not as simple as the result."

The rep had been correct: His pregnancy tests were a lot cheaper than the ones given by doctors. The real issue was the reaction of the patients. Jack was beginning to realise exactly what a "consultation" was. Some situations were perhaps better suited to the privacy of a surgery and a doctor's experience.

Good news was its own messenger. He didn't need to refer those who were happy to be pregnant; they referred themselves. After all, a false positive was unlikely, plus Jack could be emphatic with his advice: "You must see your doctor. Take this result with you."

The problem was the bad news—the unwelcome positives. They were orphans. Every patient asked the same question: "Are you sure?"

Strangely enough, the negative results, whether welcome or not, also brought their own issues. Again, the question was asked: "Are you sure?" And this led to more questions. How late was the period? Sometimes it wasn't late at all. There was unprotected sex last weekend. The period wasn't due for a while yet. They just wanted to know, to be sure

There was the problem. When Jack dispensed a prescription, he was never asked, "Are you sure?" The words "If you like, we can do another test next week or perhaps go and see your doctor" didn't carry the same ring of conviction as "These are antibiotics. Take one three times daily after food and finish the whole course."

Jack was beginning to realise the difference between dispensing and diagnosing. It wasn't that he couldn't do the test properly or that it wasn't reliable. The delivery of the result gave rise to a different set of responsibilities.

That day had begun bright and hot. Jack couldn't afford air conditioning, so the back and front doors were left open to catch a draft. Only the flies had energy.

The two girls arrived in the afternoon. The heat was still building. One was in her mid-20s and wore a work uniform. She had the sample jar. Jack recognised her; she had been in the day before, looking for the jar. The other was a teenager. She wore a uniform too.

Jack did the test. It was positive. The name on the jar was Diana. He called her in.

"Oh, it's not for me. It's Rachael's," she said.

"Who's Rachael?"

"Hang on. I'll get her for you." She went out, and Jack heard: "He says it's positive. He's inside. I'm late for work and have to go. Here's the money. Go on inside and see him. Call me later."

Rachael came in. Her hand was in front of her, offering the fiver to Jack. The school uniform was too small, a hand-me-down perhaps. Its jacket sleeve ran up the outstretched arm and scrunched at her shoulder. The news hadn't sunk in yet. She just said the words: "Are you sure?" ●

AIDS Becomes Reality for an Intern

Anonymous, PharmD

My most memorable experience happened while I was working as a pharmacy technician in a chain drugstore during my last year of pharmacy school.

In the early 1990s, AIDS to me was a subject of classroom discussion but little else. One day at work, a well-dressed man in his late 20s walked up to the counter. He looked like he was going to start crying at any moment. He was only a few years older than me. He handed me a stack of prescriptions and asked, "What is wrong with me?" I looked at the prescriptions and immediately knew from the drug names that he had AIDS. I asked him whether the doctor had discussed any of these medications with him. He said the doctor wrote the prescriptions and refused to discuss them before hurriedly leaving the room. I told him he really needed to have this conversation with the doctor and not a pharmacy technician. He pressed me to answer his question. I stood my ground because I did not want to be the one to disclose that kind of diagnosis to anyone. It was a lot of pressure for a technician. I told him we would get his prescriptions ready as soon as we could.

He eventually walked away from the prescription area and started crying as he did so. Even though this happened 15 years ago, it seems like it was just last month. •

Ethics in Daily Practice

Kathleen J. Cross, PharmD

I received a call from a pharmacy student who was conducting a survey of pharmacists. I agreed to help her out and took her survey. One of her questions had to do with ethics.

It was then that I was reminded of a young man who used to come to my pharmacy when I was a new pharmacist. Every 16 days this young man called the pharmacy to request a refill of his pain medication, and every 16 days the technician called the doctor for a refill and then complained when the doctor authorized it. The pharmacy manager would mumble under his breath and make uncomplimentary comments about the doctor continuing to refill this young man's medication.

I watched this go on for a while, until one day when the young man came into the pharmacy with a new prescription. I stopped and took a long look at his history of taking the medication. Then, I took a big deep breath, picked up the prescription, and walked over to him in the waiting area. I told him that I did not feel comfortable continuing to fill the prescription because one of the components could damage his liver with long-term and excessive use. I suggested that he seek a second opinion or maybe some alternative therapies. He looked up at me and said he had never been told that before, and he took his prescription and left.

Of course, the pharmacy manager was shocked and he was certain our next call would be from the corporate office. That call never came and the issue was forgotten.

Approximately 2 years later, I was working the weekend shift when a young man walked up to the pharmacy counter. He asked me whether I recognized him, but I did not. He told me his name, and I immediately realized who he was. I told him I had not recognized him because he had lost a lot of weight. He then told me that he had taken my advice and had sought a second opinion. He had received steroid injections in his back and had since been able to work and run and exercise. He reached across the counter to shake my hand and tell me, "Thank you."

As pharmacists, we face many challenges. One of the hardest is the challenge of balancing what is right against what others expect us to do—to keep the peace so to speak. We do not want to make waves or go against our colleagues. However, in letting someone else control our practice ethics, we lose our ability to do right by our patients. And after all, aren't they the reason we are pharmacists? ●

The Walker

Anonymous

Wakefield, Massachusetts, was one of those communities with a small-town feel located next to a modern highway. My early memories of Wakefield are from glimpses taken from a faded green Studebaker station wagon. As my family drove past, I always tried to view the beautiful lake that ended near the center of town.

I always wanted to stop and explore this town. Years later, as a pharmacy student working for a drugstore chain, I got my chance. The regional supervisor called me and said he had a store in Wakefield that needed some part-time tech help on Fridays for a few weeks.

The first week was interesting, but it was the second week that made a lasting impression. It was early evening, the pharmacy was caught up, and the doctors' offices were closed. The pharmacist and I were standing near the cash register facing the entrance when we noticed a gentleman coming toward us. He was in his late 30s or early 40s, laboring, two steps at a time, with a walker. I felt sorry for him having to work so hard to get to the pharmacy counter.

The pharmacist reviewed his written prescription and said, "I'll have to call the office for verification, if you don't mind waiting." The gentleman signaled he wanted the prescription back. Taking back the prescription, he thanked the pharmacist, turned around, and walked out, carrying the walker by his side at a fairly good pace.

When I asked the pharmacist what it was about the prescription that made him want to verify, he was silent, leaving it as a teaching point for me to figure out. ●

Identity Crisis

Fintan Moore, BSc(Pharm)

There are times when I wish that the mantra "Ask your pharmacist" could be replaced by "Send a written request, then wait by the telephone. Don't ring us. We'll ring you." Picture the following: You're not having a bad day. No mistakes in your deliveries. All your paperwork is under control. You've had a few of your nice customers in. Nobody has phoned to sell you insurance/Web sites/directory listings/mobile phones. You've just made yourself a mug of tea, and all is well in the world.

Then, one of your staff approaches to say, "There's a woman outside wants to speak to the pharmacist." You stir yourself into action and head for the counter. The lady in question has a stony look in her eyes, her lips are tightly pursed, and she is radiating cold fury. (Radiating cold is impossible in theory, but an angry woman can do it at will.) She draws you to a discreet corner, produces a tablet from her pocket, and hands it to you with the words "I found this, and I want to know what it is."

"Where did you find it?"

"I can't say."

You can immediately deduce several things without even looking at the tablet. The woman has a teenage daughter. The tablet was found in the teenage daughter's bedroom. The tablet is The Pill. The woman knows it is The Pill and just needs you to confirm the fact before burning her daughter at the stake.

To buy yourself some time, you take the tablet into the dispensary to "check a reference book." The woman has given you only one solitary tablet, which she has pressed out of its blister pack, but identifying which brand it is takes you all of 5 seconds.

You are now faced with two dilemmas, one metaphysical and the other ethical. The metaphysical one is your desire to be in a different universe many light-years away. Having failed at that, you then ponder the ethical problem. Is it a breach of patient confidentiality to reveal the identity of a medication to anyone other than the patient? If the mother had used the phrase "This tablet is my

---

Originally published in the *Irish Pharmacist*. Adapted with permission from GreenCross Publishing.

daughter's—what is it?" then I imagine you would be obliged not to identify it. But in this case, she hasn't revealed where the tablet originated and has no intention of saying until she knows what it is.

So, as the community's acknowledged expert on pharmaceuticals, how can you refuse to give information about a medication? And let's face it—the woman will find out *somehow*. All she has to do is go home and look up the telephone number of the manufacturer. The only thing you will achieve by making it more difficult for her to identify the drug is to make her even more angry.

Then, the question becomes how exactly do you tell her? There's no way to sugarcoat the pill if you'll pardon the pun. The resulting conversation will be roughly as follows:

"I've checked out the tablet, and it's an oral contraceptive."

"The Pill?"

"Well … yes."

"I'll kill her."

"I beg your pardon?"

"I found that in my daughter's room. I'll kill her."

The daughter had probably hidden the tablets in an unmarked bag behind a water pipe under a floorboard beneath the carpet, but some mothers have a way of finding things. Especially things they don't want to find.

Having confirmed her suspicions as gently as possible, there isn't a lot you can do to improve the situation. Observations such as "It's better that she's taking precautions" or "Sure, they're all at it these days" will not get you very far. Likewise, cheerfully announcing "Well, it looks like you won't be a grandmother for another while" is not the best approach.

When the woman has left the shop to go home and fine-tune her frenzied outrage, you gratefully return to your mug of tea. It's now cold. You turn on the kettle to discover that it's empty. You fill the kettle and wait for it to boil. While you wait, one of your staff approaches with invoice in hand saying, "They've completely messed up that order we gave the rep. I can't make head or tail of it." You take the proffered invoice, and you can see at a glance that a dozen phone calls to "Customer Service" lie ahead. When the kettle boils, you wet the teabag. You're out of milk. The telephone rings and a voice asks, "Can I speak to whoever looks after your accounts payable please?"

Normality has resumed. ●

Creating the Illusion

Julian Judge, MPSI, BSc(Pharm), Dip Grad Psych

Jack had seen it over and over again. It was always the same. Young men with vacant stares, swaying at the counter through an unwashed look. Their skin always gave them away. There was that something about it. It had a darkness, an uncared-for coat of mould. It was like dishwater. They were addicts but with a difference.

Forged prescriptions are easier to deal with than real ones. If you feel up to it, the best way out is to just tear it up and give it back. The key is to get the message sent: "No forged scripts here." Jack had only done that once, but it had felt great.

You can do your civic duty and call the guards. Watch while the addict sits there calmly awaiting democracy (in your dreams) whilst your customers and staff get scared. You can justify this scenario, the first few times, but as the abuse, intimidation, fear, and above all the wasted time build up, you realise that the best solution is to just avoid the situation.

So, reluctantly, pragmatically, fearfully, in fact any adverb you want, you fall back on the most reliable: "I'm sorry, we don't have any of that" or "I dispensed the last one this morning. I'm really sorry; I should be getting more in tomorrow, but you never know." Then you pick up the phone and ring your local pharmacies: "Sorry to bother you, but we've just had a forged script." It's a cop-out, yes, but you justify it based on a whole lot of reasons. They all distill down to one thing: Send the message "Don't bring forged scripts here."

However, as mentioned previously, these were addicts with a difference: They had genuine scripts. It's now the land of the surreal as Mr. Joe, whose forged scripts (yes, that's plural, not a typo) you are tired of seeing, suddenly has an endless supply of the genuine article: always the same doctor, always the same drugs, always the same dosages, always the same quantities. Beautiful, crisp, just paid for, shiny prescriptions are presented to you for your professional dispensing. And it's not only Mr. Joe, but it's his friends too, and Joe's a popular guy. He has a lot of friends, and they all have crisp, shiny, just paid for, white pieces of professional paper.

Originally published in the *Irish Pharmacist*. Adapted with permission from GreenCross Publishing.

Every single one has the exact same items, dosages, and quantity. You professionally reflect as you realise that you have never seen a script for anything else from this doctor—no antibiotics, inhalers, blood pressure medications, nothing. You ring this land of vapour and enquire, to be told, "That's right, and if he gives you any trouble, send him straight back to me."

You make discrete enquiries of other professional prescribers and dispensers and realise that, "No it's not just you; it's everybody." So, you ring your Society and present them with your dilemma. They're sorry for your troubles, but there's nothing they can do: "You'll have to make a report to the Medical Council." You reflect on this, and then you consider the implication of commercial suicide.

But the question still stands. You know these patients have been changing doctors, forging prescriptions, jumping all over the city from Jack to Jill, and yet they suddenly have this brand new supply route—and they want a prompt professional dispensing service from you.

So, you're back to the old reliable: "I'm really sorry. We're all out of this today. Try tomorrow. I'll have some in then." Yes, this does present the distinct actuality that the drugs will get dispensed somewhere else, but you have a distinct problem. Unless you stop this, your little local community pharmacy will quickly turn into a black hole of fear and lost custom. That's your ethical problem. Deal with it as you will, but here's Jack's story.

Initially, the "We don't have them; I'm terribly sorry" line was working, but when the forged scripts became real ones, the clientele were a little more reluctant to accept their hard luck. That's where Pat the Magic Man helped Jack.

The Magic Man was there one morning and witnessed Jack try to persuade Mr. Joe that "I am all out of these again." It went on a while until Mr. Joe, shouting expletives, yelled, "You're full of … I'll get the bus to … They always have them there." "That's inspiring," thought Jack as he watched the door slam.

"You know, Jack, you're not creating the illusion," Pat said as he smiled. "I'm sure you have your own reasons for not wanting to give that, eh, young man what he wants. And that's all very well. But, you see, here's the thing. He doesn't believe you. And I don't believe you either. It's not enough to tell him you haven't got them; you've got to show him. That's the main trick to magic: Show, don't tell. Then he'll believe you."

Jack replied, "Educate me, Pat."

"Show me what he wants," Pat said.

Jack produced a fairly full tub of diazepam five. Pat opened it, whistled a slow note, and said, "Look at all those little juices. Problem is, they've got yesterday written all over them. There's still something to be said for a pint. It's like … how shall I put it? Awe. Yes, let's use that word. Awe. A fresh pint—it's got an organic feel to it. You don't get that colour of black in anywhere else." Pat spread his hands apart as if addressing the Roman Senate.

"Anytime I get a pint of the Black, I'm in awe. But Jack! I digress. Excuse me, but it's a favourite subject of mine. Now, where was I? Oh yes—creating an illusion. You see this here tub? Well, empty it and leave it somewhere very prominent. Don't open and show it to him, but rather let his eyes find it. People do notice things, you know, especially when they want something. Well, let him find it. That way, you've given him hope and expectation. Give it to him. Let him open it. Then, he'll believe you." ●

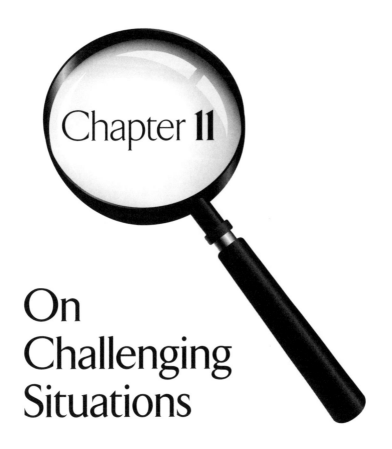

Chapter 11

On Challenging Situations

The ultimate measure of a man is not where he stands in moments of comfort and convenience, but where he stands at times of challenge and controversy.

—Martin Luther King Jr.

Hurricane Katrina: Pharmacists Making a Difference

Jef Bratberg, PharmD, BCPS

The New Orleans Hornets basketball arena floor smelled of heat, sweat, and doom. Fire alarms were still screaming, albeit in an ever-decreasing frequency and pitch, as their strobes called for attention that wasn't going to arrive. The only constant source of light was red exit signs around the ring of the arena. Two Disaster Medical Assistance Team (DMAT) tents, surrounded by dozens of black Federal Emergency Management Agency (FEMA) tote boxes, were barely visible at one end of the arena. Opposite the loading dock entrance sat abandoned DMAT sport utility vehicles (SUVs), 3 feet of dark brown floodwater lapping at the loading dock beyond. My DMAT team surrounded the commander and listened to his message: The patients we would see were suffering from disorders exacerbated from stress and lack of drugs for 5 days....

My first mission as a disaster pharmacist had begun.

A Team Forms

I completed my deployment prerequisites for the Rhode Island DMAT (RI-1 DMAT), a part of the National Disaster Medical System under FEMA and the Department of Homeland Security, in the summer of 2004. The team was activated for Hurricane Frances that summer, but I was unable to participate because of my employment commitments at the University of Rhode Island College of Pharmacy.

In the summer of 2005, I advanced my disaster training at the team's biggest event—the Rhode Island National Guard Air Show. I met and worked with many teammates who were to become my Gulf Coast "family."

In late August, chief pharmacist Megan Sliney and I met at the DMAT office to discuss drug inventory and management. Although August was one of our team's three on-call months, head nurse Lori Tucker joked that day that no disaster could happen the next weekend—two members of the team were getting married! On that gorgeous Saturday, my mother called to ask if I were going to be

Originally published in the *Journal of the American Pharmacists Association*, 2005;45(6):654–8. Reprinted with permission.

activated for Hurricane Katrina, a Category 1 hurricane that had caused minor damage after making its first landfall in southern Florida. I found this unlikely because I would have been already called up if it were truly severe.

The next morning, I woke up to polish fall semester lectures for the infectious diseases courses I teach. After glancing at the CNN Web site and learning that Katrina had reached Category 4 status, I knew the telephone would soon be ringing. Lori called first, and I asked if Megan was going to go; she said yes. But after thinking about my many obligations at the university, I declined her invitation for this mission. I was just too busy to participate.

However, after a few minutes of thought, I changed my mind, and I was promptly placed on the FEMA roster. I learned that the team was leaving very early the next day, and I hadn't even started packing. In the next 16 hours, as Hurricane Katrina reached Category 5 status, I bought hip waders, assembled my gear, and completed the essentials for my classes until my kind department chair picked me up at 5 am to drop me off at the airport. I began the physical and emotional journey of a lifetime.

Hurry Up and Wait

As the team winged its way to Alabama, Hurricane Katrina, with 145 mph winds, made its second landfall, this time near the mouth of Louisiana's Pearl River. Coastal communities were obliterated by the storm's power, and low-lying areas became a part of the ocean. The storm surge swamped parts of New Orleans immediately, sending residents to their roofs, and breaches formed in the levees protecting New Orleans, which would soon essentially be part of Lake Pontchartrain, flowing and ebbing with the tides.

By the time we met in Anniston, Ala., on Monday afternoon with several team members who had arrived the prior day, Katrina was making its third and final landfall near Pearlington, Miss. On Tuesday we packed up and convoyed to Camp Shelby, Miss., with the intent of deploying to devastated Biloxi. Federal law enforcement officers escorted our SUVs and three FEMA trucks through a Mississippi night made darker by lack of power in 80% of the state and more dangerous by pines that had reached skyward a few hours earlier but were now lying on the ground a few feet from the highway.

At 5 am on Wednesday morning, we arrived at Camp Shelby and collapsed in the early morning heat at its former World War II prisoner-of-war barracks. We ate military meals ready-to-eat (MREs) and experienced refreshing cold showers. We waited for orders. Whoever put Baton Rouge in the betting pool won because that night we drove there past checkpoints and signs reading "I-10 Closed," "New Orleans Closed," and "Emergency Personnel Only." After arriving at Louisiana State University (LSU), we rested for a few hours on a gymnasium floor.

I will never forget watching that Thursday morning as a continuous stream of military helicopters arrived to drop off critically ill patients, presumably plucked from New Orleans rooftops. The overall activity was overwhelming—volunteers of every sort, including many LSU students, helping in every way. Megan and I helped the U.S. Public Health Service pharmacists dispense medications in the gymnasium hospital. I even remember that a volunteer physician accepted an IV–PO antibiotic switch recommendation. Even in disasters, interventions can still be made!

Watching televised reports of New Orleans descending into chaos, we anxiously awaited orders along with DMAT teams from across the country. Finally ours came: Go to the causeway to set up our hospital and provide medical care for thousands of people stranded there. Because of safety concerns in the increasingly dangerous New Orleans, we later were reassigned to the mission of a lifetime: Deploy to the basketball arena next to the Superdome and provide badly needed medical care for the remaining 6,000 evacuees who had been holed up for days in hellish conditions at the Superdome.

Its roof ripped away by Katrina's winds, the Superdome was a wreck, with water in its underground parking garages and human waste and in fact remains in its hallways. Nearby stood a Hyatt hotel, its windows blown out by the storm as proof that vertical evacuation was not enough. Both structures stood as symbols of the inadequacy of the emergency plans laid out for New Orleans. Like the levees, these structures perhaps could have withstood a Category 3 hurricane, but Katrina provided more than they could handle.

Our team's strong leadership successfully argued that the team should not deploy until both the indefensible causeway and the Superdome were secured by thousands of Army troops. We also wrangled 12 Federal Protective Service officers to guard our 35-person team (6 officers per 12-hour shift).

We went to bed with two instructions: don't shave because any cuts could provide entry for bacteria from the floodwaters, and because of security issues, pack only items that you are comfortable never seeing again—just in case we had to "bug out" as the previous team had. I chose food over my camera and cell phone (which had no signal anyway), one set of clean clothes, took my last hot shower for a long time, and slept on a mattress.

We're Here to Help

As many Americans rested up for a lazy Labor Day weekend, we were awakened that Friday morning at 4 am. Once we assembled the convoy, we hit the road under escort, driving through intersections without stopping until we reached

Interstate 10. Our first destination was the New Orleans airport, where we would leave our vehicles and hear from an assessment team about conditions at the Superdome.

The airport was truly a war zone. If I thought helicopters were landing frequently at LSU, that stream paled in comparison with the activity at the airport. Helicopters from every armed service delivered human cargo like bees dispensing pollen at the hive. The noise was deafening, and the number of people with body armor and large weapons outnumbered those without.

We boarded passenger vans thinking about the advice and insights provided by the assessment team ("the bathrooms are bad but not any worse than the worst gas station restroom"). Soon we were in New Orleans, the same city where 4 years earlier I started the process of joining the faculty at the University of Rhode Island during a Midyear Clinical Meeting of the American Society of Health-System Pharmacists. Despite the high level of security and assurances from my team commander, it was difficult to feel safe. I felt for my Leatherman knife more than once, wondering if I would need to use it.

We drove past a burning chemical plant on the Mississippi River and the wind-damaged downtown that spewed black smoke into the bright summer morning. Then I saw the people: people who had lost everything, drinking bottled water and eating scraps of food on freeway ramps and bridges around the Superdome, people who before had simply appeared as television images but were now giving us an inspirational thumbs-up. A new hope ran through me: we were here to help, and these people were happy to see us.

We drove down the exit ramp to the flooded streets surrounding the Superdome, moving past an abandoned DMAT van poking out of the water. The driver revved the engines and gunned the van to the arena's loading dock, nearly sputtering out when water splashed across the hood and against the back of the van. We made it. We were here.

Our priority was to enter the pharmacy, which looked like a well-stocked disaster itself. The pharmacy also looked like a scene from a ghost town: a half-filled amber bottle on a half-written FEMA prescription, awaiting its label and final check, greeted us inside. For the first 4 hours, I can't truly recall what I did, with my dehydration and caffeine-withdrawal headache exacerbating the heat, humidity, and the odor of human waste.

Good news—we didn't have to unpack our drugs! I had always hated checking in orders and other inventory tasks in the pharmacy. Thanks to the Oklahoma and New Mexico teams who were forced to abandon their drug caches, we would not need to unpack and transport dozens of pharmacy totes up several flights of dark, slippery steps. However, Megan and I still had to sort everything and evaluate our quantities, posting three sheets of paper on the wall with duct tape (a lifesaver, especially in a disaster) that listed all the medications.

Memories to Last a Lifetime

Our team was thus lucky to have double the drugs available during our weekend at the Hornets Arena. We were also fortunate to have two community- and FEMA pharmaceutical cache-experienced pharmacists to operate the pharmacy and improve its organization.

Megan Sliney worked the first night shift. Per the DMAT motto, "Eat when there's food, drink when there's water, sleep when you can," I wandered down the dim, putrid maze of hallways and stairs, lit only by fluorescent tubes, to the VIP lounge/DMAT rest area. I placed my baby wipes, knife, eyeglasses, and deodorant on a small table in a booth and laid down to rest. I awoke around 7 am and returned to the pharmacy to relieve Megan. While she slept, I continued to organize the pharmacy, placing suspensions in one area, injectables in another, narcotics hidden in the back on boxes of diapers. We had boxes of injectable antibiotics, plenty of tetanus shots and insulin, albuterol inhalers, antibiotic ointment, and antifungal creams. I wrote labels and filled scripts for 5 days of drugs for patients evacuated from the Superdome and/or by helicopter. This policy was exasperating for both the prescriber and me, as we had no idea where the patients were going to go, and whether they would be able to get medication there! We also struggled with dispensing to military personnel who were deployed without medications. We did what we could, and they were grateful.

I remember counseling a gentleman who likely lost his eye after getting stabbed in his socket while trying to board one of the buses leaving the Superdome. We gave him a few Vicodin, and I could see that he was still in pain while waiting for alternate transportation. I showed him my handwritten label on the bottle and said that he could take two now. He shook his head and said, "These pills are all I've got. I'm going to save them."

On that morning after sleeping in the lounge, I was working in the pharmacy when suddenly I was told by other team members to shut and lock the door: shots had been fired outside, and we were locking down and performing accountability. I could open the door only for people who knew the password. After the "all clear," three people who had been shooting at helicopters were dead, and the survivor was treated at our hospital—stat cefazolin IV.

We dispensed all kinds of medications while deployed at the arena. Megan made a phenytoin admixture one night for a man experiencing intractable seizures. When our mental health professional asked what psych drugs we had, I told him haloperidol, fluoxetine, and nortriptyline. We dispensed haloperidol for all psych patients who had depleted or lost their antipsychotic agents—and the federal cache wasn't designed to refill primary care prescriptions. The funniest request of our pharmacy was for Depo-Provera—for one of the reservists!

In our off time, we bleached the floor, rearranged cots, exchanged soiled cots for clean ones, dined on MREs, and marveled at our surroundings. At our door, I'll never forget the image of two police officers, personifying the definition of absolute exhaustion. They had been on duty for 5 days straight, but they only slept occasionally in their car; they were out of food and gas, and their radios were dead air. They said, "Thanks for being here," and we evaluated and treated them and then offered them a clean, dry cot for as long they needed one.

We stayed true to our motto: "RI-1 DMAT—We're there when you need us."

Beyond the Call of Duty

According to our patient files, our team treated more than 160 patients in just over 48 hours. Megan and I did more than dispense prescriptions; we organized, moved, and reset the pharmacy; guarded our supply of antidiarrheal medication and narcotics; and recommended treatments for a chronic obstructive pulmonary disease exacerbation from our limited formulary. Disaster pharmacists must indeed be resourceful. Yet even in these most dire of circumstances, we upheld key tenets of the Oath of the Pharmacist: making the welfare of humanity and relief of human suffering our primary concerns and applying our knowledge, experience, and skills to the best of our ability to ensure optimal drug therapy outcomes for the patients we served.

Pedialyte was one of the more common requests processed by our pharmacy, and we had quickly depleted all the stock left by the other DMATs. I knew that we had to break into RI-1's drug cache. With the pharmacy under constant, close supervision by our "samurais," the Federal Police Service "ICE" guys, I asked our logistics chief, Mark Palla, about getting into the "Refer" (the refrigerated truck) to get some Pedialyte from our cache. When Mark opened the back door of the "Refer," cool air blasted me. He rearranged some boxes and held the top of the cardboard tri-wall containing our pharmacy cache (minus narcotics) while I examined the red pharmacy totes. They still had their tie-downs attached, so with flashlight in teeth and knife in hand, I jumped into the tri-wall, cut the ties, tossed the flavored bottles of Pedialyte into the cramped walkway of the truck, and relieved Mark of the burden of holding the plastic cover of the tri-wall. Then I had to throw the bottles into a hand truck and carry them up the multiple flights of cement stairs covered in body fluids and slippery diesel fuel to reach the pharmacy.

And I used to hate inventory day at the pharmacy. ●

Daytime Drama

Janet Bradshaw, BSP

Some events stick in your mind forever. I never looked forward to working on Sundays. Even though it was only a 4-hour shift, it just seemed that all hell was going to break loose when I was working alone. Little did I know what I was in for one particular Sunday.

On this day, things were relatively calm. The phones were ringing off the hook as we prepared to open the store, but that was nothing unusual. One of our front-store staff, a high school student, came up to me in the dispensary some time later. In her calm, soft voice, she asked whether I knew where Dan was. Dan is one of our pharmacists, a single guy, who lives out of town and pretty much keeps to himself. When I indicated that I had no idea where he might be and questioned why she was asking, she replied, still in that quiet tone of voice, "The transplant coordinator is on the line; they have a kidney for him but can't reach him." I almost fainted.

Dan had gone on the transplant list just a couple of months before. Nobody, least of all him, expected that a kidney would come up this quickly. As a potential recipient, he had to supply the coordinator with four contact numbers. Apparently, this person had been trying to reach him for a couple of hours already and was not successful. She was not amused.

Time was of the essence. I quickly sent this young girl to check on his place. Neither of us knew exactly where he lived and had no clear direction except to head west to the end of the lake. I think by now she realized the seriousness of the call and was probably more than a little scared of what she might find.

I started calling his neighbors—no luck getting hold of anyone. Knowing I needed help, I contacted a couple of staff members, who in turn started phoning people who might have seen him at his local hangouts—the coffee shop, a friend in a neighboring town, his mom's place. And, nothing.

Our young staff member was gone for a long time. That worried me, too. When she came back, she was shaking. She relayed that the neighbors had seen him leave that morning but knew nothing more. Poor thing had pounded on his door, thinking the worst. By now, we had exhausted our attempts to find him. His mother had driven out from the city and was beside herself with worry.

I decided to call the police as a last ditch attempt. In the meantime, I had a call from the transplant coordinator, who was more than angry. When I asked whether we could do something to help, she replied that it was the patient's responsibility to maintain contact with the coordinator at all times; if that wasn't the case, then tough luck—the kidney goes to someone else. I explained that we had the police out searching, when all of sudden, I got a frantic message from another staff member that the police wanted to talk to me on the other line.

OK, my plan was to buy some time with the coordinator and in turn hear what the RCMP (Royal Canadian Mounted Police) had to say. They were asking me some routine questions, and she was telling me that essentially he had run out of time and was being passed over for this kidney. At that, I could have cried as my boss walked in and I handed one phone over to him.

All of a sudden, I heard, "They found him!" Sure enough, he had gone to the city and was on his way home. He decided to charge his cell phone, but for some reason, it turned off. He was somewhat annoyed when he was pulled over by the police, but his attitude changed quickly when they asked, "Are you waiting for a kidney? Well, there is one waiting for you. Come with us!"

At that point, we were all shaking but relieved, and I couldn't have been happier as I relayed the news to the coordinator. Still miffed, she agreed to give him the kidney provided he got there pronto. There was still a 3-hour drive to the city. Dan was so visibly shaken that my boss drove him to the city. The surgery went well.

It has been 1 year since that date. It is still so fresh in my mind that it drains me in reliving it. This scenario could very well have been a script written for a TV drama.

I should mention that to add to the stress the computer system in the entire store crashed while we were trying to find Dan. Thank goodness, one of our managers, who was also involved with the "hunt," came speeding in when she received my SOS and worked to restore the system. For some mysterious reason, the usual deluge of patrons did not appear while the search was on. Help from above, perhaps? ●

Per Una X o S (For X or S)

Giorgio Tosolini

A young couple wearing colorful clothing, obviously foreigners, entered the drugstore in Italy. The junior pharmacist, who was helping them, read the prescription and asked her manager for assistance. She gave him a medical prescription that was on green paper, an unusual color. It was issued by the Andalusian Ministry of Health in Spain.

The couple spoke mainly in Spanish because their Italian was poor, but they were able to inform the pharmacist that they were temporarily in Italy and that the medicine was for their 1-year-old daughter, who had a thyroid condition.

The handwritten prescription read, "Levotirosina sol. 20 mcg/ml," but the medication was not listed on the Italian computer database. The pharmacist prudently asked for more time to research it, and they consented.

At the end of the day, after closing the drugstore, the pharmacist began his research on Google. He couldn't find much information on *levotirosina* at first, but the search suggested a similar term, *levotiroxina*, for which many links were provided, primarily in Spanish. He also found some publications in which both terms seemed to be used interchangeably. The pharmacist—because of his naiveté or just because he was tired—assumed that the two substances were the same. Some years ago, this wouldn't have happened to him. But now he is busy with prices, discounts, receipts, copies, and so on. It appears that someone has decided to kill his job slowly and has succeeded.

To get more information about *levotirosina* (levo-tyrosine), the pharmacist wrote to an Internet forum but without success. The next day, he called a drug company and was able to talk to someone who was familiar with *levotiroxina* (levothyroxine). The company's representative cautioned him about the stability of the drug in water and about the dose, which seemed excessive for a 1-year-old child. The scrupulous pharmacist called another supplier who had in his listing sodium levo-tyrosine. This supplier told him that the substance dissolves well at the concentration given in the prescription. It didn't occur to anyone that the substances might have been different.

The next day, the young couple returned to the drugstore. The pharmacist advised them to consult a local pediatrician to monitor their daughter's therapy.

The father guaranteed that he would do so but insisted on having at least one prescription of levothyroxine to temporarily continue the child's care because they had run out of the medication. Considering that it was difficult to find a doctor on a Saturday, the pharmacist conceded and gave them the medication, recommending that they be careful with the dose. They left, leaving the prescription on the counter, which was then filed.

That day, a relative visited the pharmacist. Responsible for a chemical analysis lab, she was an expert analyst. As they discussed what the pharmacist had found out previously about the discrepancy in the solution and stability of the drug, the analyst realized that the first supplier with whom the pharmacist had spoken was talking about levothyroxine and the second about levo-tyrosine. She explained to the pharmacist that both substances, although metabolic precursors of each other, are completely different. One, levo-tyrosine, is an amino acid, and the other, levothyroxine, is a hormone. Levo-tyrosine is used to treat phenylketonuria, which is caused by an inability to metabolize phenylalanine to tyrosine, and levothyroxine is used to treat hypothyroidism. She also encouraged him to check the PubChem Web site, which clearly explains the two different structural formulas.

Anguished, he ran to the pharmacy to review the prescription. It was handwritten, but there was no doubt—it was an S, not an X.

But why had the couple talked about the little girl's thyroid problem? Was there a misunderstanding because of the language barrier? Maybe the girl had a different illness.

The pharmacist immediately consulted his primary physician. "If the little girl has a thyroid problem," he said, "you were right in what you gave her." However, the pharmacist wasn't sure that the girl had a thyroid problem. He had to find the couple and correct the situation. The dosage of the medicine he gave them was nontoxic if taken for a short time, but the parents could administer the wrong treatment for a long time.

But where could they be found? He had only their last name. On the Internet, he found the name of the pediatrician who wrote the prescription. A medical roster showed that the doctor was in Cordoba, Spain, but there was no address. The pharmacist spent an unforgettably long Saturday and Sunday alone in his pharmacy. He contacted the Spanish embassy in Italy for help, but they gave him only a cellular number because, they explained, they must protect the privacy of the people he was looking for. That was all they could do for him. Then, he called the Italian embassy, but nobody answered the phone. So, he decided to write an e-mail to the embassy, but the address was inactive. By Sunday evening, after a frustrating day, he told a friend about the situation. His friend remarked that the patient's last name sounded like it was from Romania.

This small tip led the pharmacist to the Roma camp near his town, where he was well known and welcome. Their numerous children had grown up wearing his children's clothes and shoes, sleeping in his children's crib, and playing with his children's toys. The camp's oldest man came forward, and the pharmacist got confirmation that the last name on the prescription was a Roma name. However, the old man did not know the young couple. At that point, the pharmacist headed for the police department, where he explained the situation. There, finally, he found help.

The police told him that the family lived in a nearby town, 7 miles from his drugstore. The couple didn't have a permanent phone, so the pharmacist immediately drove to their home. When he arrived, he saw laundry hanging out to dry in the yard and a long line of shoes of all different colors and sizes at the doorstep, suggesting the presence of many children. He finally found the young couple but didn't want to alarm them. He told them that he just needed to review the little girl's medical documentation to verify the therapy. They invited him into their kitchen and gave him a pile of Spanish medical references and typed green prescriptions. He was able to verify that the girl had hypothyroidism, and so *levotiroxina*, with an X, was the correct medication.

The only wrong prescription was the one carefully handwritten by the Cordoba doctor. ●

How I Saved a Patient's Legs

Fred J. Pane, BPharm

I was director of pharmacy at a 250-bed community hospital. An infectious disease (ID) physician approached me to order a nonformulary anti-infective to treat an infection in both legs of a patient. He said if the infection wasn't cured, the patient was going to have both legs amputated below the knee.

I reviewed the patient's chart and saw that he had been in the hospital four times in the past 6 months with oozing wounds in the back of his knees (he didn't manage his care well at home). The notes stated that if the wounds did not begin healing, the surgeon would proceed with the amputations. I went to see the patient, and we discussed his medical history (surprisingly, he was not diabetic). He told me that all he wanted was to keep his legs so he could take his granddaughter ice fishing.

I ran an idea by the ID physician about using nitroglycerin (NTG) ointment topically around the wound to try to increase blood flow and, ultimately, antibiotic tissue concentrations. The ID physician said if the cardiologist had no problem, we could try it in combination with the nonformulary anti-infective. The cardiologist gave his approval, and about 30 minutes before each dose of anti-infective, a nurse applied about one-quarter inch of NTG ointment above the patient's wounds.

The wounds began to get better and finally healed, perhaps because of the improvement in circulation from the NTG and better anti-infective penetration. The patient was discharged, and I began to see him taking walks around the local area.

One day, the patient showed up at the hospital to present the ID physician, his internal medicine physician, and me with clocks that he made. I have hung that clock on the walls of my offices and at my house. It is a reminder that we need to think outside the box in patient treatment and that we can have an impact on patient care. ●

Farmaco Urgente (Urgent Drug)

Giorgio Tosolini

In Italy, as elsewhere, we have vacation days and holidays, and lucky are the ones who can enjoy them. Unfortunately, sick people stay sick even at Christmas and New Year's. One of my patients is a very impatient old man. He is always in a bad mood, and usually I don't like to attend to him.

One holiday, after waiting his turn, the man came forward and demanded, "Doctor, you must give me an antibiotic." Very politely I asked him, "What kind of problems do you have?" It was obvious that he was suffering, and he whispered that he had not been sleeping and felt an unbearable burning sensation and constant need to urinate.

I explained to him that his symptoms were serious and that he ought to see his doctor. He said that his doctor was on vacation and that his substitute couldn't be found anywhere because of the holiday. On rare occasions, I do give patients medication without a doctor's prescription, which is legal in Italy. (The patient still has the responsibility to see a doctor within 24 to 48 hours. A delayed diagnosis can be a big burden for the pharmacist.) However, I remembered that this patient was seriously ill, but I couldn't remember what he had.

People were lined up and pressing to be served, so I just gave him the phone number of an after-hours medical service, even though I knew it would be hard for him to get in touch with the service. I told him that he could also go to the emergency room, which was always crowded and involved a long wait.

He went away angry, but he came back in the afternoon. I asked, "Well, sir, how did it go? Did you find a doctor?" Surprisingly, he handed me a prescription for an ultrasound test. I told him that he surely had another letter containing the prescription for a medication. "Yes," he whispered. "But it's in a closed envelope!" He had left the envelope in his car. He went to get it, and upon returning, he gave it to me.

I went directly to the bottom of the paper, where the prescription information is usually located, and saw "Bactrim DS," an antibiotic. I thought to myself that because he had a minor illness, maybe it wasn't worth making him spend half a day in the emergency room. But then, just above the prescription, I noticed "Relapse of prostatic neoplasia. I advise a chemotherapy cycle with …" I gave him the medication and also advised him to take the letter to his doctor the next day in order to start the treatment as soon as possible. He paid and, as always, left quickly without saying goodbye. He forgot the letter on the counter. I ran after him and repeated, "Don't forget the letter, and take it with you to your family doctor!" Annoyed, he answered, "Yes, yes, okay," and walked away. ●

A Day in the Life of an Inpatient Pharmacist

Darrell Hulisz, PharmD

Pharmacists are ideal professionals for ensuring that the medication reconciliation process is properly executed at every point of service. In my early years rounding on a general medicine ward, I had a firsthand experience that confirmed the important role that pharmacists fill in taking an accurate and complete medication history.

It was a Monday morning in July. I was pre-rounding when I came across a 46-year-old woman admitted over the weekend with fatigue, nausea, vomiting, myalgias, and bruising. She was previously in good health, with the exception of chronic low back pain secondary to a herniated lumbar disc for which she reported taking occasional acetaminophen as needed. Other than mild back pain, she reported periodic leg cramps, neuropathic in nature, likely secondary to her lumbar disc disease. However, on admission, she had a new onset of extreme fatigue, hemolytic anemia, low platelets, and a serum creatinine of 4.2 mg/dL. She had no prior history of blood disorders or renal disease.

During rounds, one of the interns asked the patient whether she used any other medications, and she said no. During this patient's first 48 hours of admission, a battery of lab tests and imaging studies were conducted, and a renal biopsy was scheduled to determine the etiology of her new-onset renal failure, hemolysis, and thrombocytopenia. Later that afternoon, I did what had become my routine, namely, interviewing all newly admitted patients to obtain a detailed medication history, probing for the use of over-the-counter medications and dietary supplements. I asked the woman whether she ever took medication to help her leg cramps. At that point, she told me that she occasionally took 260-mg quinine sulfate tablets, though for some reason, she hadn't disclosed this to anyone else. Was it because no one asked specifically about her use of over-the-counter medications? Did she believe quinine was not important enough to mention? Perhaps she did mention it, but it was not reported by any of her caregivers.

I vaguely remembered that quinine was associated with platelet dysfunction, although I needed to do a literature search to satisfy my curiosity. Sure enough, I found four isolated, but confirmed, case reports of hemolytic–uremic syndrome associated with the use of quinine. The clinical and pathological features, onset, and lab findings were strikingly similar to those of our patient. I searched for someone on my team to report this to. Better still, I ran into the consulting nephrologist. With copies of the case reports, I somewhat timidly made a recommendation to consider a test for quinine-dependent platelet antibodies. (I only knew about this test after reading the case reports.)

The next morning, the residents and attending on our service thought I was a genius for making this "discovery." However, I was only doing my job—that is, simply taking a good medication history and posing the question of an iatrogenic disorder.

The patient's renal function continued to deteriorate, and she developed a pancytopenia. She was treated aggressively, and fortunately, she made a reasonably good recovery. Incidentally, her test for quinine-dependent platelet antibodies came back positive, which confirmed quinine as the likely etiology of her hemolytic–uremic syndrome.

Although it has been many years since I encountered this patient, I can recall numerous times when I, another pharmacist, a pharmacy student, or a resident made similar discoveries. Pharmacists are uniquely trained to conduct detailed and complete medication histories, including drugs used as needed, over-the-counter medications, vitamins, herbs, and dietary supplements, along with the specific dose and dosing schedule for each. Pharmacists can readily identify incorrect dosages, possible interactions, and potentially inappropriate drugs; discover drug allergies; and uncover potential adherence problems. The contribution of the pharmacist extends well beyond obtaining this history. It also often includes making specific recommendations to improve patient care outcomes in a variety of possible scenarios and pharmacy practice settings. ●

Sweet Taste of Trouble

Fintan Moore, BSc(Pharm)

In spite of several years working as a pharmacist, it was only on becoming a parent that I realised the importance of children's medicine tasting as pleasant as possible. Dealing with a sick child is bad enough without having to force-feed spoonfuls of yucky-tasting liquid every few hours. Some children have incredible "antibiotic resistance" and will only take their 5-mL dose when their arms are pinned by one parent while the other parent squirts it down their throat with a syringe. Life is so much easier when a child likes the taste of medicine and looks forward to it as a tasty little treat. This can, of course, have its drawbacks.

My daughter has just turned 3 years old and quite enjoys the taste of "pink juice" (paracetamol [acetaminophen]) and of "white juice" (ibuprofen). She looks on enviously whenever her 1-year-old little brother is getting either medication, and she would happily grow a few more teeth if she thought it would get her a few spoonfuls. She has also grasped the concept that if something is wrong with her, then she might get one of her favourite coloured juices.

One night every week, my wife works late, which leaves me as a solo parent for the bedtime routine. Like most men, this situation stretches me to the limit of my ability to cope. Women's brains are definitely wired better to watch more than one child while simultaneously managing other tasks—that's my excuse and I'm sticking to it.

During one recent lone-parent evening as I was running a bath for my two kids, my daughter said, "Daddy, I've a sore tummy. I want pink juice." She then disappeared from the bathroom. I was busy taking off her brother's clothes and didn't give her tummy any more thought. Having taken off his nappy, I was about to pop him in the bath, but the water was too hot to put him in, so I ran the cold tap. He took advantage of the delay to crawl out to the landing and pee on the floor.

Having spotted the puddle and mopped it up with the nearest towel, I tucked him under my arm and wondered where his sister had gone. I found her in his room putting what was left of a bottle of paracetamol back on its shelf. One of her parents hadn't replaced the cap properly, so it hadn't been as childproof as it

Originally published in the *Irish Pharmacist*. Adapted with permission from GreenCross Publishing.

should have been. The portion missing from the bottle was distributed among her clothes, the duvet, and, presumably, her tummy.

The 140-mL bottle was about a third full, but I didn't know how much had been in it when she took off the cap. I did know that a child has to drink a lot of paracetamol before coming to harm, so I asked her calmly "How much of the pink juice did you drink?"

"Lots." Not the answer I had hoped for.

I placed her brother on the floor and rang Crumlin Children's Hospital while leafing through some reference data on paracetamol. The lady at the hospital advised me to bring her in. As I hung up the phone, I was grateful that her brother was still dry. Then I heard the splash as she dropped him into the bath! I still don't know how she managed to lift him over the edge.

I had found the toxic dose of paracetamol: 150 mg/kg body weight. After fishing her brother out of the tub and wrapping him in a towel, I led her to the weighing scales, which naturally gave a reading in pounds. So, I drove to the hospital, trying to mentally convert pounds to kilos and multiply by 150. My daughter was unhelpfully breaking my concentration by repeatedly telling me, "I only little. I not know how to take a little bit."

The hospital waiting room was full; however, the triage nurse saw us almost immediately. She measured the remainder of the paracetamol in the bottle at 45 mL. Given the benefit of a pen, paper, calculator, and metric weighing scales, she was quickly able to confirm that even if my daughter had drunk the entire missing 95 mL, she was under the toxic level, and I could safely bring her home.

Having lectured her about only mummies and daddies being allowed to give medicine, I got her ready for bed. I turned out her light and was about to leave her room when she whispered, "Daddy, I was only pretending."

"You mean, you didn't have a sore tummy?"

"No, I didn't." And she hasn't had one since. ●

The Whales: A Pharmacist's Story

William R. Wills, RPh, FIACP

There I sat, a common ordinary pharmacist, on Saturday, May 26, 2007, waiting for a combined group of renowned scientists to arrive at the Rio Vista Coast Guard Station in Rio Vista, California. I was delivering the second package of antibiotics that I had compounded to save (or at least improve) the life of two patients. This was nothing new for me, for this is what I do on a daily basis: improve the life of a patient or (as innumerable letters attest) save the life of a loved one. What made this experience so different from the rest? The patients were so big! The daughter weighed an estimated 12,500 pounds and the mother was an estimated 55,000 pounds, and they drew a large amount of attention. These patients were also big news scientifically, because this was the first time that whales in the wild would be injected with antibiotics. We were honored to be part of a historic experience.

Whale Tracking

Delta and Dawn, as they had been dubbed, were mother and daughter humpback whales. They had been featured in the news for 17 continuous days since they were first sighted on May 10. They were sidetracked on their journey north to Oregon, and for some reason, they came into the San Francisco Bay and traveled north up the Sacramento River Delta, where they became stranded. Some have theorized that the whales had an infection that impaired their navigation. To escape, they would have to travel almost 100 miles south. Their senses couldn't process that task, because it was the opposite of their instinctive behavior. As a result, they were stranded in fresh water, which is foreign to their skin and other body systems and was causing their general health to deteriorate. These problems were exacerbated because both whales had injuries that weren't healing. Although those injuries, which appeared to have been made by a propeller of a ship, were not life-threatening, they added another insult that had to be overcome by the patients in a time of crisis.

Originally published in the *International Journal of Pharmaceutical Compounding*, 2007;11(5):376–83. Reprinted with permission.

For 17 days, hundreds of people had been involved in the monitoring, health care, and navigation of the whales. Some of the government and volunteer agencies that joined the effort were:

○ Alaska Whale Foundation
○ Marine Mammal Center (Sausalito, California)
○ National Marine Fisheries Service
○ National Oceanic and Atmospheric Administration
○ U.S. Coast Guard

Efforts were made to get the whales to turn around and return to their natural habitat (the Pacific Ocean); whale song that was broadcast over speakers did not alter the situation; boats had been positioned to prevent the whales from going farther upstream; and at one time, 26 boats unsuccessfully tried the pipe-banging method to get the whales to turn around. Rough water and winds gusting up to 20 miles per hour hampered attempts to attach a global positioning system (a satellite-monitoring device) to the mother's fin.

Our Pharmacy's Role

Why was I at this event? Which great thing that justified my being part of the lifesaving team had I done? Nothing that my staff or I had done was extraordinary; we were called upon to do what we do every day. What makes our pharmacy different from most pharmacies, however, is that we are a compounding pharmacy that concentrates on trying to meet the unique needs of the individual patient. Although most of us may never have the opportunity to treat patients as large as whales, we can make a whale of a difference (pardon the pun) in the lives of those around us and in our business. So what brought this singular experience to Grandpa's Compounding Pharmacy, a "compounding only" pharmacy in a small town in northern California?

May 24, 2007, was a normal Thursday for our pharmacy:

○ Patients were coming in to see if we knew of other options that their regular pharmacy or doctor hadn't thought of to solve their unique medical challenges.
○ New prescriptions that required new formulations were being prepared and checked.
○ Refills were being prepared.
○ Patients were picking up their medications.

○ Patients were being counseled about how to take their medications and what to expect from new medications.

○ Consultations with physicians about new alternative treatments were being conducted.

Then there was the phone call that we received at 4:20 pm from a pharmacist in Orange County, which is about 450 miles from our pharmacy. He was inquiring about whether we could (or would) prepare a particular antibiotic to be given by injection. After he had told me what the medication was (a trimethoprim and sulfamethoxazole combination), I felt comfortable about preparing the compound, because we had done so in the past. However, I wondered why a pharmacist so far away wanted me to prepare a medication for one of his patients. I was told that Sea World had contacted that pharmacy about preparing the medication. However, the pharmacy's regular compounding pharmacist was on a 2-week vacation (the first vacation in 8 years), and the fill-in pharmacist did not feel qualified to prepare that particular complicated formula. The medication was for two whales somewhere in Northern California that were injured. We considered the whales "ours" because we had been following their progress for more than 2 weeks on every major news network, and we knew that they were not far from us. Although we knew that we could compound the medication, we did not have enough of the necessary ingredients to prepare a sufficient amount of the formulation for such large mammals. It was late in the day, and I didn't know if we could still schedule a next-day delivery. If we missed the next-day delivery deadline, then because of the Memorial Day holiday, the soonest delivery would be Wednesday of the following week. I said that I would check with our supplier in Houston, Texas, to see if there would be time to place and receive an order. The Orange County pharmacist was concerned that if we purchased the ingredients without a written prescription (which neither pharmacy had received), we would incur an unnecessary expense and might be stuck with an inventory of medicine that we would not be able to use. I reassured him that in no way would I want him to feel guilty if that happened, but I insisted that the medication be ordered immediately to ensure our chances of helping the whales. Twenty minutes after ordering the medication, I received a call from a veterinarian at Sea World who furnished me with a prescription. If I hadn't ordered the ingredients when I did, we would have been past the cutoff time for next-day delivery.

In the meantime, Frances Gulland, Vet. MB, MRCVS, PhD, the chief veterinarian at the Marine Mammal Center, who was working with the veterinarians at Sea World to treat the whales, contacted me to confirm that we would be able to compound the requested medication in the right quantity and dose and to discuss other aspects of the treatment. All of us were then on the same page.

Thursday night, a local television station featured a story about our preparing the medication. Everybody was excited about our involvement in the efforts to help the whales. As expected from "Grandpa Extraordinaire," I contacted my posterity (10 children and 46 grandchildren) and some friends to alert them about the broadcast.

I anticipated the arrival of the trimethoprim and sulfamethoxazole on Friday morning, May 25, and our plan of action included:

- ○ Dry sterilize one of the powders (a 3-hour process).
- ○ Sterilize the other powder by making it into a clear solution and running it through a sterilization filter (a 1-hour process for a total preparation time of 4 hours).
- ○ Personally deliver the medication to a courier in Sacramento who would take the medication to the Rio Vista Coast Guard Station.

If all went well, the whales would receive their medication Friday evening, May 25.

On Friday morning, all our staff members were excited as they performed their regular duties. My time was being taken up with the media and further communication with the veterinarians, who contacted another drug company to see if a second specific antibiotic (enrofloxacin) could be obtained to prepare a concentrated suspension for injection. That was indeed possible, and I was then given prescriptions for doses of 3 mg/kg for the 25,000-kg cow (Delta) and the 5,000-kg calf (Dawn) at a final concentration of 333 mg/mL of sterile injectable preparation. The cow's dose was 187 mL, and the calf's dose was 40 mL, but the darts for injection would only hold about 60 mL each. I was asked whether I could prepare that medication also. After researching the preparation and talking to some consultants, I felt that I could prepare an acceptable sterile injectable suspension. The drug company promised that a formulator from their staff would call and would work with me to develop a good formula. The formulator never called, so I had to draw upon all my training in compounding, use my best judgment and the special equipment that we owned, and be a true compounding pharmacist. The soonest that the drug company could ship the enrofloxacin active pharmaceutical ingredient in bulk was that evening (if they put it directly on a plane), which would set back our original Friday deadline for the administration of the medication to the whales. Fortunately, we received a reprieve: The first and second antibiotic compounds did not have to be ready for administration by the afternoon, because the "shooters" (the people who would actually be shooting the medications into the patients) wouldn't arrive from the East Coast until late Friday evening. Therefore, the shooters couldn't be on the water until early Saturday morning. We would have until 4:00 am on Saturday, May 26, to get it all done. We would then hand-deliver the medication to the Whale Operations Command Center in the Rio Vista Coast Guard Station.

The first antibiotics (trimethoprim and sulfamethoxazole) didn't arrive until about 3:00 pm on Friday. This meant that the preparation wouldn't come out of the dry sterilization procedure until 6:00 pm. Darci and Nick, two of our certified technicians who were working that day, volunteered to stay until that antibiotic preparation was finished. A short time later, a television crew arrived to do another story, and Darci and Nick were spotlighted on television, which they really deserved because they didn't go home until 10:00 pm that evening. At 9:00 pm, Dan, another of our certified technicians, picked up the enrofloxacin at the airport. He took the drug to the pharmacy laboratory, and I began to work on it immediately to get it as concentrated as possible. Other challenges that we faced were working with a large quantity (250 g) of powder and the need to maintain sterility. Finally, at midnight, I prepared a medication that appeared ready for administration. I called the veterinarian, Felicia Nutter, DVM, PhD, to find out how large a needle would be used to inject the material. She happened to have the shooter in the car with her when I called, and he provided that information. Even though the concentration was thick, it went through the needle. It was then time to package the medication into individual vials, seal it, and place it into the sonicator (a special device that keeps suspended material in small particles). I left the pharmacy at 2:00 am, and Dan stayed to monitor the sonicator function and to ensure that the preparations remained in suspension. I returned at 4:00 am to perform a final check of the medications and to gather supplies.

Saturday morning, my sweetheart and I first met the people with whom I had been communicating over the phone. They are a good group; down to business but gracious and courteous. I worked with the shooters to help fill the darts with the antibiotics. We were able to insert the enrofloxacin into the first darts without a problem. However, the second set had crystallized in the containers because it was too concentrated. I gathered up the medications, left the trimethoprim/sulfamethoxazole with the doctors to use back at their facility, and took the enrofloxacin back to the pharmacy laboratory in Placerville. I called Jill, the laboratory technician with the drug company, and told her what had happened and what I had done. Unfortunately, she was not a formulating technician and had no suggestions other than providing a key bit of information about the pH. The drug manufacturer usually has to keep the pH at 11 when they are working with this medication, but the literature that I had been working from stated only that the pH had been adjusted. With that tidbit of information, I adjusted the pH of all the compounds, reliquified the medication, and put the compounds in the refrigerator until their delivery on Monday morning. Sunday, on the way home from church, I stopped to see how the preparations were doing. They had become semisolid, and that wasn't good. I had three thoughts about how to fix that problem, and I decided to use the idea about which I felt the strongest. I mixed the material from syringe to syringe and found that the preparation was about the consistency of yogurt, which is smooth and would easily pass through the needle. I then transferred all the medications to syringes and planned to show the veterinarians and shooters how to mix the medication between two syringes on site. That procedure enabled the placement of the medicine directly into the darts. Even though the water was rough and the whales were moving that day, the shooter was able to hit both whales easily (and at the site he had chosen) with the first darts of enrofloxacin. The veterinarians were well pleased.

The veterinarians, who had found some information stating that the trimethoprim and sulfamethoxazole might crystallize in the tissue of the whales, decided to not give it and to let the whales rest and just observed their movement and general disposition. On Sunday, the whales were acting much less lethargic, and their skin looked better.

On Monday morning, I gave what was left of the enrofloxacin to the chief veterinarian at the Command Center and showed her how to mix the preparation from syringe to syringe so that it could be used for a final injection. That was when we discovered that the whales had traveled downstream. The veterinarian and her team took the remaining antibiotics back to the Marine Mammal Center to use experimentally on other injured patients. My job was done.

The darts were an interesting device. The barrel, which contained the antibiotic, was a hollow aluminum tube about 15 inches long. The needle, which was about 8 to 10 inches long, was a hollow stainless steel tube with a pointed end. Just below the shoulder, where the point was formed, were four holes on the four sides of the shaft, and the medication was released through those holes. The needle screwed onto the barrel, and the medication was put into the other end of the barrel. A plunger was inserted, all the air was forced out the needle end, and the barrel was sealed on the back end. Over the holes in the needle was a band that fit tightly so that none of the medication was released before the needle was shot into the animal and the medication was forced into the tissues. The tube was then pressurized with air to 130 pounds of pressure that drove the medication into the animal. After the darts had been filled and assembled, they were taken out onto the boat and were shot from a rifle that was a modified .22 caliber.

Conclusion

Here is another question that we have been asked: "Since there are other compounders in northern California who have the special license needed to make sterile injectable medications, why did they call you?" The answers are logical: The pharmacist who called our pharmacy (1) had been (and still is) associated with us in promoting good-quality compounding, (2) belongs to the same organizations to which I belong, (3) had consulted with us about various issues from time to time, and, simply put, (4) knew us. He knew that he could depend on us, that we would do a good job and not let him down, and that the consumer would be pleased with our service. We know that we can count on each other, and our integrity is intact.

Skin scrapings taken from the whales on several occasions during their time in the Sacramento River revealed that they are from the Eastern North Pacific stock of humpback whales. Analysis of the mitochondrial deoxyribonucleic acid of the scrapings confirmed that the calf is a female. It is good news that this endangered species is reproducing.

The whales were last seen on Wednesday, May 30, 2007, just outside the Golden Gate Bridge. They were heading farther out into the Pacific Ocean and have not been seen since. Once again, we have (perhaps) saved and have definitely improved some lives through compounding. Many people have expressed their appreciation for what we did, because they were rooting for the whales. We are so blessed every day to be able to work with physicians of all kinds to help humans and animals by providing individualized, customized medications that control pain, restore quality of life through hormone therapy, ensure the comfort of the dying, decrease anxiety, help a child swallow a lifesaving medication, prepare a medication that can be applied topically, and much more! ●

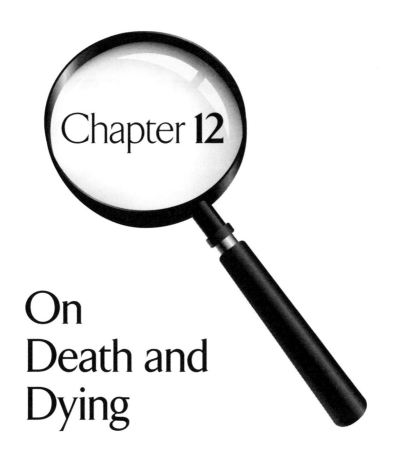

Chapter 12

On Death and Dying

To cure sometimes, to relieve often,
to comfort always.

—Anonymous

Kathryn

Joanna Maudlin Pangilinan, PharmD, BCOP

I could hear the smile in her voice—not the pain, fear, or loneliness.

"Hi Joanna. How are my numbers today?"

It was a familiar routine. Kathryn was calling the pharmacist-run anticoagulation phone clinic for her results and dosing recommendations.

"Hey Kathryn! You're a little high. Have you been eating OK this past week?"

Our typical patient had received a hip or knee replacement and was referred to us for short-term warfarin therapy. Kathryn wasn't our typical patient. She had had a sinosagittal thrombosis years ago and was one of our few long-term warfarin patients.

I had never laid eyes on Kathryn. I didn't "know" her from her chart, either, but from our past year of telephone exchanges. She had been fighting genitourinary cancer since she was in her mid-20s. Now 20 years later, it was closing its grip on her life. You could almost tell from her anticoagulation. Her international normalized ratio, or INR, was continuously high despite the smallest of doses of warfarin.

"Yes, I've been eating OK. I try to drink supplements when I can, and I actually had a nice seafood dinner the other day."

Eating, or lack thereof, has a dramatic effect on patients' tolerability (vulnerability?) to warfarin. I always suggested consistency. But really, by this time, Kathryn was probably more knowledgeable about warfarin and eating than I was. Was consistency even possible for her?

"I just want to confirm what dose of warfarin you have been taking since we last talked."

Her dosing had been pretty consistent until recently. However, it wasn't the warfarin dosing that I found difficult. It was the voice that had been conversing with me over the past year. That beautiful voice that had told me about her disappointment in not being able to date or get married because of her condition. That beautiful voice that had told me about being self-conscious and nervous about leaving her house or having people visit her. That beautiful voice that had expressed great happiness for me when I told her I had met "the one" and was getting married.

"I've been taking 1 mg every other day. But I think I vomited my dose on Saturday."

Being a caretaker for Kathryn weighed on me heavily. Her condition was very serious, and she seemed to be getting worse. Her eyesight was now failing. Those beautiful eyes I hoped viewed all happy sights and not a counter cluttered by extended- and immediate-release morphine. How much can a person take?

"Go ahead and take 1 mg tonight. Then take 1 mg on Tuesday and Wednesday. Can you get another blood draw on Thursday?"

Kathryn told me she was bleeding continuously and being transfused almost every week. A call to her oncologist confirmed my suspicion: It was time to stop warfarin. After her oncologist discontinued the warfarin, we dismantled her anticoagulation chart. It hadn't been my intention to get Kathryn discharged from our service. Days later, she was placed on hospice. Her mother called asking who they should turn to for medical care now that everyone left them.

"Sure, Thursday is fine. I'll talk to you then."

I assured her mother that her oncologists would still take care of her. We were still here, too. No one was leaving her. I continued to call Kathryn once in a while. Her beautiful voice had a chord of melancholy. Her hopes changed to regrets.

"Sounds great! Have a good few days, Kathryn."

Kathryn died the week before my wedding. Although we never met, I will never forget her beautiful voice and the lessons she taught me about friendship. ●

A Hard Lesson to Learn

Jane McKimens Adams, MS, RPh

I grew up in a drugstore. My father was the pharmacist and owner of one of two drugstores in our small town of 1,500 people in southeast Kansas. As such, he was one of the pillars of the community, although he would never think of himself that way. Quiet and unassuming, never looking for the spotlight, he just went about his business caring for the health care needs of the people of our town and doing his part as a local businessman to support the community at large. He even pulled a part-time stint at the local 20-bed hospital so that it could have a pharmacist on site each morning to review orders and set up medications. Needless to say, I thought his were large shoes to fill when I decided to pursue pharmacy as a career.

Once I started professional studies, though, I found out there was a lot more to pharmacy than the community store in which I grew up. My coursework in clinical pharmacy and an elective in hospital pharmacy introduced me to all sorts of opportunities to carve a different niche for myself in the evolving field that is pharmacy. By the end of my final year in school, I had already accepted a position in the teaching hospital where I did clinical rotations. No small-town druggist's life for me, I was going to be a hospital pharmacist in a big city!

I eventually went on to pursue graduate work in the field, having moved even farther from my hometown to Texas, where I studied for my master's degree in hospital pharmacy. After graduate school, I stayed in Texas, working in a hospital that was building on the growing trend of decentralized, clinical pharmacists. It was exciting, rewarding, and demanding, and I knew that my skills were being used and tested every day. Only once did I go back to my hometown to work in my father's store, when he was recovering from surgery and was instructed to stay in bed for a week. I knew he would appreciate not having to pay a relief pharmacist, so I arranged to be his relief for that short period of time.

Within a couple of years, he retired, and I no longer had the opportunity to offer him that particular gift again. He then worked part-time for his former competitor, who had become the owner of the only remaining drugstore, but my father responded to the community as if he were still its full-time "druggist." Dad took the phone calls at home from the hospital and the nursing home, delivering medications that the doctors called in after hours. For the patients who called to say they couldn't get to the store before closing time, he would go back to meet them at the store so they could start their medication that evening. When the owner wouldn't answer his home phone, they called my father. Like I said, he was a pillar and as dependable as they come.

It was after one such emergency delivery to the nursing home that my father came home and complained of a nagging chest pain that just wouldn't go away. The frigid December air of that Christmas morning certainly didn't help, but my mother knew it was more than the cold air, and she made my father go to the hospital to get checked out. They ran the usual electrocardiogram and blood tests, not finding anything abnormal, but kept him overnight for observation "just in case." In the wee hours of the next morning, he had a cardiopulmonary event from which they couldn't resuscitate him, and he passed away. When that phone call came at 4:30 in the morning, I knew before answering that it wasn't good news. It almost never is at that hour, is it?

After the shock of his sudden death, I went through many emotions. My first reaction was guilt: Why did I have to be working that Christmas and not be with my family? My next reaction was anger with the small-town hospital: Did the staff really know what they were doing in the middle of the night? How many times have they revived someone who was "coding"? If only he had been in a larger, more progressive hospital, I told myself, the outcome would have been different. I clung to that thought, even though my sister told me they had done everything they could, and nothing worked. She was there in the middle of the night—I was second-guessing them long distance.

A few short weeks later, I was working a decentralized position in my large teaching hospital, when a code blue was called for one of my assigned units. Rushing to the patient's room, I quickly assumed my role as the pharmacist on the code team. I prepared medications that were ordered, helped monitor the patient's responses and the time between doses of medications, and anticipated the next medication that might be ordered according to the guidelines for advanced cardiac life support I had learned. The team followed all the appropriate algorithms, but the patient didn't respond to anything we did. After some time, I heard the attending physician say, "I'm afraid we have a pulmonary embolism here," with the unspoken thought that there was no way we could get him to surgery to treat it in time. And at that moment, the decision was made to stop resuscitation efforts and let the man go peacefully.

Once the code ended and I was able to leave the patient's room, the parallel of that situation with my own father's clinical situation hit me like a freight train. Being on the team that followed all the guidelines and still couldn't successfully revive that patient, I was given a powerful reminder that there are some things we just cannot control, no matter how large the hospital or experienced the team. That realization brought me the peace I needed to accept my father's passing as one beyond reach of human talents, but it also taught me a valuable lesson in professional humility. ●

The Unanswered Plea

Kathryn L. Hahn, PharmD, DAAPM

I had just begun working in a community pharmacy setting after 10 years in an oncology/pain/hospice hospital setting. I was trained in inpatient pain management and had thoughts of translating that into the community setting but was so busy with the change of work skills required that it had taken a back burner.

During the second year of my new practice, I received a wedding invitation from a close friend. While attending the wedding, I became acquainted with the father of the bride. I took a particular interest in him because he had chronic pain. We sat at a quiet table at the rehearsal dinner, and he told me his story.

"I have had numerous back surgeries, but none of them have helped the pain. The doctors say they can do nothing more for me, so I just get my bottle of hydrocodone and acetaminophen each month, which now doesn't even take the edge off. I can't live like this anymore," he explained.

"Have you tried to see a pain specialist, or ask for a referral?" I asked in alarm. "If you can't find anyone in your area, I can help you find one in mine."

"I'll think about it," he said, before he was pulled away by dinner guests.

I later asked the bride, a registered nurse (RN), what she knew of her father's condition, and she said, "He likes his pain pills a little too much. Yes, he has back pain, but our family thinks he'd be better off not taking long-term narcotics for it."

I made sure the bride's father had my e-mail address and telephone number before I left and thought of him occasionally once back home.

Approximately 6 months later, I got a call from my RN friend, who said, "My dad passed away last week. He took the entire contents of his pain medication bottle just after picking it up. He was in a hepatic coma for 3 days and then passed away. It was tragic, but we feel it was for the best—he was in so much pain."

Now, I help health care professionals become better educated about what addiction is and is not, learning that "relief-seeking" is different from "drug-seeking" and that pain does kill. I pray that through education, we can reduce the occurrence of patients with pain wishing to end it all because they can't find a provider who will help lift them from the hell they live in. ●

Paracetamol

Julian Judge, MPSI, BSc(Pharm), Dip Grad Psych

June 1, 1985, came early that morning with heat. Hospital 4 rang. They wanted Carbomix (activated charcoal), fast. "Quickly please, it's urgent!" This was a hospital pharmacy. Drug requests were routine, but this was the first time one was urgent. Normally, drugs were requested by a nurse, reading steadily off a chart, but this voice was angry and frustrated.

Jack had just started a 6-month contract with the hospital. His official start time was 9 am, but he quickly learned to get there at about 8. That way, he could solve problems before they built up. This hospital was one of Dublin's largest. Its pharmacy department was very different from the shop where he had done his prerequisites, and Jack knew that he had a lot to learn.

For the first few weeks, he was assigned to hospital 2, which was mainly a geriatric ward. Things happened at a reasonable pace, and provided he had his *BNF* (*British National Formulary*) available, he was in control. Patients there were established, and the twice-daily drug-trolley chart check proceeded at a steady but not demanding pace. Then, he was transferred to hospital 4.

Hospital 4 was the reserve ward for accident and emergency admissions. Jack enjoyed it. It had a buzz—an edge—that other wards lacked, plus there was Willa. It was set in an old Victorian part of the main hospital. The brickwork was red, floors wooden and scrubbed, ceilings high, and acoustics sharp. You could hear shoes click. Sometimes Jack would tap his heel while walking to get a beat. That's how he met Willa. He, in his own world, was flicking his heels to get a click as he walked—a morning tap dance.

"Hey girls, it's Fred Astaire. Do that again." He looked up to see a set of crossed eyebrows with a hint of smile. "Well Mr. Tap Dancer, you must be our new pharmacist. I'm Willa."

Hepatocellular necrosis is the major toxic effect of paracetamol (acetaminophen) poisoning. Biochemical evidence of maximal damage may not be apparent until 72 to 90 hours after overdose.

Originally published in the *Irish Pharmacist*. Adapted with permission from GreenCross Publishing.

Emily was 17 and had just been admitted. Jack never got to see her, but throughout that week, he heard her story, mainly through Willa.

Any patient should be considered at risk of severe liver damage if he or she has ingested more than 150 mg paracetamol/kg of body weight, or in adults, more than 12 g (24 standard tablets), whichever is smaller.

Emily had taken at least 60 tablets of paracetamol. No one really knew for sure. She was unconscious when they found her. All her parents knew was that they found various packets of paracetamol in quantities of 12 and 24 beside her. Some were old; some were not. Price tags revealed various sources, mainly a supermarket. Why had she taken them? There were various answers. Basically, she thought she was unloved, unwanted by friends, unable to cope. She had been doing her high school graduation exams. There was pressure. Did she mean to do herself harm? Unlikely, especially given her response when she regained consciousness.

Patients who present 15 hours or longer after ingestion are more difficult to treat and are at greater risk of developing serious liver damage.

No one knew exactly when she took them. Her family was away for the weekend. They found her on the Monday morning they returned home.

Though the benefit has not been demonstrated, administration of 50 g of activated charcoal may be considered if given within 1 hour of overdose.

It was an exercise in futility, but Jack's Carbomix was given that morning. It had a dull black ditch water look about it, but there was not one person in hospital 4 that week who would not have gladly taken it for her if it would have done any good.

Individuals who have overdosed on paracetamol have no specific symptoms for the first 24 hours. Although nausea and vomiting may occur initially, these symptoms in general resolve after several hours. After resolution of these symptoms, individuals tend to feel better or may believe the worst is over.

Emily was unconscious when she was admitted that morning. She regained consciousness sometime that evening, and by all accounts was lucid. Word must have spread throughout that week of what she had done. Willa told Jack she had never seen so many young visitors, most of them girls in school uniforms. Basically, Emily regained consciousness, and everybody she "thought didn't care" came to visit. Irony is vicious, but, effectively, they were saying goodbye. Emily had regained enough consciousness to relate what she had done and why she had done it. She then had the rest of the week to understand what she had done and to say goodbye.

If a toxic dose was absorbed, after this brief feeling of relative wellness, the individual develops overt hepatic failure.

As the week progressed, hospital 4's mood went down. Everybody was crying. Jack didn't know much about liver transplants, but there were no fresh liver donations that week.

Massive hepatic necrosis leads to hepatic failure, renal failure, cerebral oedema, sepsis, multi-organ failure, and death within hours.

Emily had taken a lot. Some people overdose slowly by taking maybe two or three tablets above the maximum dose for a long period of time. Then, they take a second drug, which also contains paracetamol, but they don't know that.

That's why paracetamol shouldn't be sold in supermarkets. Years later, when arranging his over-the-counter medication shelves and regarding what should stay behind the counter, Jack often thought of Emily. ●

Gerald

Pamela Stewart-Kuhn, RPh, MPA, CGP

H e was an ordinary man with an extraordinary soul. Like many of the military
retirees I served at the pharmacy, he preferred to use the base pharmacy.
I think many of them like to hold onto that last remaining link to their time of
military service. He was elderly, and I suspected he was at a point in his life where
he had been retired now for longer than he had actually spent in service. We
never discussed his military career, so perhaps he preferred to live in the present.

Gerald had an uncanny knack for showing up in the pharmacy waiting
room when we had just closed the window for lunchtime or on the afternoons
we were closed for training. He never complained—just patiently sat waiting for
the pharmacy to open. If he had been rude or impatient, I probably would have
gone about the business of eating my lunch and catching up on my paperwork.
However, his calm, sweet demeanor always led me to ask whether he needed
something, despite the lunch hour.

He was kind and thoughtful, and in the spring, he picked us blueberries from
the many bushes in his yard. I could tell he took the same thoughtful, patient
manner with something as simple as picking blueberries. There was never a
branch or unripe berry to be found in the bags he brought us.

Over the months, we would chat for a few minutes each time he came in, and
I learned about his wife Josie. She had late-stage Alzheimer's disease and resided
in a local nursing home. He told me how every day he would go and have lunch
with Josie. He knew that most days she didn't know who he was, but he returned
day after day to the nursing home. Sometimes he would have breakfast with her
as well, and he would sit with her and hold her hand. Never once did he show any
signs of self-pity or regret that would seem so natural under the circumstances. He
told me how he loved his Josie now more than ever—he loved her even more than
when they were first married.

One morning in October, on one of his visits to the pharmacy, he told me
that he had to go in for heart surgery. Fortunately, he would be able to recover in
the same nursing home as Josie. I never saw him again. Several months passed,
and I realized that he hadn't come back. I called the local nursing home to inquire
about him. The nurse told me that Gerald had "expired" the day after his heart

surgery. I never found out what became of Josie. I imagine that if she's still alive, he's still there with her, holding her hand, waiting patiently for her to join him.

We live in a society of instant gratification and disposable relationships. Most people don't believe in the existence of an everlasting, romantic love, and few ever experience it. Because of Gerald, I know it's real. ●

I'm Afraid of Dying

Doreen Pon, PharmD, BCOP

She was a 40-something Filipino woman. That morning, she was sitting by the window in her hospital room when I came in to check on her patient-controlled analgesia pump. We talked a little bit about her pain medications, and then she grabbed my hand and whispered, "What is it like to die?"

I had been an oncology pharmacist for more than 5 years, and watching my patients die and families grieve had become part of my daily routine. I felt I had developed a tough professional exterior and a pragmatic outlook on both life and death, but my patient's question caught me off guard. I felt helpless, not knowing how to answer her.

It's taken me a couple of years since then to learn that most patients don't really expect you to be able to answer. They just want someone to listen to them, to acknowledge their fears, to allow them to cry. It doesn't make it any easier for me, though, when patients and families ask me questions that I can't answer. I, like most pharmacists, have been trained as an "information person." Pharmacy school can't teach you compassion. Compassion is something I've learned from my patients. ●

Loretta

Pamela Stewart-Kuhn, RPh, MPA, CGP

She was an elderly Southern lady, sweet and soft-spoken. She had bright blue eyes and wisps of white hair around her head. She was the definition of spiritual grace, despite the circumstances of her life and her illnesses. She never complained, and she had plenty of reason to do so. She had been widowed for several years. She was facing a round of tests to rule out cancer, and she told me she had beaten colon cancer once before. She decided that if the good Lord was done with her, she would gladly join her husband. If not, then she would stay until He was ready to let her go.

Time passed, and before I knew it, almost a year had gone by. When I saw her again, I barely recognized her. Her son came in with her, pushing her in a wheelchair. In a cruel twist of fate, she had suffered a massive stroke in her brainstem but had not died. She was no longer able to open her eyes, because her muscles were paralyzed by the stroke. Despite the fact that her body was failing, she was still very lucid.

She had been in a rehabilitation facility for almost a year and was finally going home. She was delighted to be back in the pharmacy and was filled with her usual sweetness and gratitude. I gave her a hug and fought back the lump in my throat. I was shocked at her condition but figured if she wasn't full of self-pity, I shouldn't feel sorry for her either. She told me that her son had given her a cat and that "he's going to become a good friend." She lasted another 6 months or so before the Lord finally finished her time here on Earth.

Her life will always hold important lessons for me. She showed me that you can be content, and even happy, despite difficult circumstances. She was a living example of grace in the face of grave illness and great suffering. ●

Pharmacy Buddies for the Terminally Ill

Submitted by the Koninklijke Nederlandse Maatschappij ter bevordering der Pharmacie (Royal Dutch Association for the Advancement of Pharmacy)

Pharmacists Anne-Margreeth Krijger and Leonie Hulst of the Stevenshof Pharmacy in the Dutch city of Leiden wanted to improve the care their pharmacy offered to terminally ill patients. They came up with the Pharmacy Buddy Program, which couples a terminally ill patient with a team consisting of a pharmacist and a pharmacy assistant. The buddy program is both simple and effective. It shortens the lines between patient and pharmacist and contributes toward continuity of care to the patient during the final phases of life. The program also enhances contacts between pharmacists and other health care professionals. The Royal Dutch Association for the Advancement of Pharmacy awarded Stevenshof with the first prize in the 2009 Pharmaceutical Care Awards.

Continuity of Care

Anne-Margreeth: We started thinking about it after we had participated in a training program on palliative care. The teacher was very inspiring and informed us about the special needs of patients who are near the end of their lives: continuity of care and regular contact persons. The continuity of communication was said to be particularly important.

Leonie: Now, in a pharmacy such as Stevenshof, with a lot of staff members who work different hours, it was rather difficult to arrange this continuity of care. We really had to think of a completely new way of organizing the care for terminally ill patients. During a brainstorm session with members of our pharmacy team, we hit upon the idea of the buddy.

No Hassle

Anne-Margreeth: This is what we do: We team up a pharmacist and a pharmacist assistant. They will be the buddies for a patient who is terminally ill. You might say they are the *face* of our pharmacy for the patient in question. Patients as well as family caregivers always get to see the same pharmacist and pharmacist assistant. In this way, they are spared the hassle of having to explain the situation over and over again. Also, when the doctor calls to discuss the patient's medication, the call is transferred to the buddy-pharmacist who of course knows exactly what the situation of the patient in question is. Our pharmacy now has three buddy teams. The teamwork within the framework of the buddy program has also further improved relations within the pharmacy team itself. It is very rewarding to work together this way.

Doctors' Approval

Leonie: Before we started the program, we discussed it with the doctors our pharmacy is in contact with. They reacted very positively indeed. Together, we agreed upon certain guidelines. For example, when would be the best time for a patient to enter the buddy program. It is the doctor who determines this and who provides the pharmacy with the necessary information.

Anne-Margreeth: The buddies then make an appointment with the patient and, if possible, with the next of kin to explain what the buddy program entails. We have arranged for the buddies to receive special training focused on the different needs of a terminally ill patient occurring at different times during the dying process, such as wound treatment, nausea, and constipation.

VIP Treatment

Leonie: Patients who enter the buddy program get what you might call VIP treatment. When their medication runs out, they do not need to call the automatic pharmacy repeat medication telephone line but can call their buddies directly. If necessary, we also see to it that the medication is delivered to the patient's home. Often, we have known the patients for years, and we want to do the best we can for them—especially in their hour of need.

Anne-Margreeth: Since we work like this, we have much better contact with the home care organizations. Ordinarily, the work of a pharmacist begins when the doctor's prescription comes in. Now that we really know about the patient's situation, we can anticipate. For example, when a family caregiver comes in with a first-time prescription for morphine, the buddy will try to find out what the medical indication for this prescription is.

Leonie: The work is of course very intense and can be emotionally draining. We also pay attention to this aspect of the buddy program. How to protect your professionalism, and at the same time, stay involved in the patient's situation. All of us agree that the buddy program gives an extra dimension to our work at the pharmacy and we would not want to work in any other way.

Closure

Anne-Margreeth: In the final days of a patient's life, the buddies and the patient or caregiver are in daily contact. When the patient dies, there is an abrupt end to this intense cooperation. This did not feel right. Both the family of the deceased and the buddies need some sort of closure. We therefore always write a letter of condolence and offer the patient's family the possibility for a final meeting with the buddies.

Leonie: We have worked with our buddy program for a year and a half now and helped dozens of patients. Our work is very much appreciated. The other day someone told us, "Stevenshof is really *my* pharmacy!" Very rewarding indeed. ●

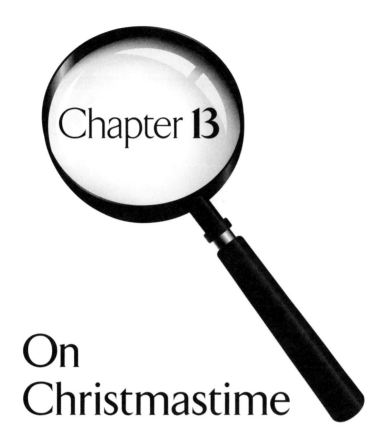

Chapter 13

On Christmastime

It is, indeed, the season of regenerated feeling–the season for kindling not merely the fire of hospitality in the hall, but the genial flame of charity in the heart.

—Washington Irving

Santa's Cure

Gary R. Anderson, RPh

Many years ago, I worked as a decentralized pharmacist in a children's hospital in St. Paul, Minnesota. It was around the Christmas holiday season, and I was covering the pediatric intensive care unit (PICU). A party with Santa was planned for the kids who could make it. For those who could not, Santa would come visit them at their beds.

A very small child who had open heart surgery a few days before the party was in the PICU. He was still hooked up to all the ventilators, IVs, pressors, diuretics, and so on and was not doing well. I watched as Santa visited this young child. He bent over the PICU bed and whispered something to the boy. I never found out what Santa said, but from that moment on, this small innocent child began his recovery. He started to get better, day by day, until he was discharged to a non-PICU bed and eventually to home.

Many medical miracles are the result of medications. I truly believe this miracle was a result of whatever Santa whispered to this young child on that day. ●

A Very Live Christmas Tree

Robert A. Lucas, PharmD

It was December 1992, and I was living in Frankfort, Kentucky, and working at a local pharmacy chain. I worked full time as a pharmacy technician while taking classes at night toward completing my prerequisites for pharmacy school.

One day, a young woman approached me at the cash register and asked whether we had anything to help with her ear pain. "I am having pain that comes and goes in my left ear," she said. I took her to the "ear" section of the store, but I wanted to get more information about her symptoms.

I didn't have to wait long, because while I was asking her for more details, she started jumping and stomping her feet like she was having a tantrum, crying and letting out muffled screams, and covering her ear with her hand. She said she felt like something was moving in her ear. "It comes and goes, and it scares me," she added.

Knowing that any medicated drops would probably not be a solution to her problem, I took her back to the storeroom, used a penlight to look in her ear, and unexpectedly found nothing. She finally gave information about when the symptoms started, stating that she was putting up her live Christmas tree and something "fell into my ear." I referred her to the emergency department at a local hospital.

Several hours later, she returned to the pharmacy to thank me for trying to help her. The emergency department team had extracted a live spider from her ear that caused her to tremble and shriek when it would intermittently move. ●

A Christmas Dream

Steve Cummings, RPh

Sometimes truth is revealed through the magical. Many years ago, the author worked at Jolly Drugs in Knightstown, Indiana. An unexpected room above the pharmacy imparted a deeper understanding of the place and people he served.

I had been working at the pharmacy part time for about 3 years the first time I walked up those stairs. It was during the busy season between Thanksgiving and Christmas. Those 30 or so days had always seemed magical to me. I was helping one of the clerks, a woman who did most of the store's merchandising, bring down extra shelves, because prescription business that morning was a little slow. She had lived around this small Indiana town all her life and was one of the reasons people came to the store. She knew everyone and their likes and dislikes. Every so often, I asked her to fill me in on the store's history. Why did the backroom still have all the old medicine bottles and a prescription counter—just the way somebody's grandfather had left it? What was that customer's secret for keeping a newlywed twinkle in her eye as she looked at her husband of 40 or so years?

The clerk had told me once before that there was a ballroom on one of the floors above the store. I could feel something—*elegance* is the best word—as we climbed those wide oak stair boards. Even the pitch of the staircase was set in a manner that would allow women in their best holiday evening dresses to enjoy their arm-in-arm stroll to the ballroom. By now, the brass key was turning in the lock's tumblers. With a nudge, the oversized door swung open.

Everywhere I could see the efforts of a day of Christmas decorating. Each gaslight on the wall was lit and had boughs of the most fragrant evergreens attached with satin ribbons of the perfect shade of Christmas red. The soft gas flame's light reflected off the highly polished dance floor and hit the many loops of gold garland hung around the ceiling, creating the twinkling of no less than a million stars in an Indiana night sky.

My sense of smell tugged, and I glanced to my left. There, on a long table, was a buffet dinner that only the women of a small-town church could have put forth. Half the table was filled with the favorite dish of each family in town. The other half had only the best of the town's pie makers. More evergreen boughs had been expertly placed here and there, along with a centerpiece of flickering Advent candles.

But where was the Christmas tree? How could I have missed it? There! In the east corner it stood by the tall windows to be viewed from the street below. Surely the noblest tree in all of this part of the world. Its many lights were small white candles set among strings of popcorn and cranberries. The decorations were paper, cut, colored, and hung by each member of the Sunday school classes. Small red velvet bows had been scattered in between, and all seemed to point to the top. A star like no other I had ever seen was there. It looked like it had been created from the thinnest sheets of brass, and it reflected every possible ray of the candles' light.

That newlywed's twinkle! That was it! That was how all those years of happiness had started. It was the memories of times past and thoughts of sharing times to come that made it last.

Oh, the stories a room can tell you. Have I been born in the wrong time? No, I don't think so. Yet, there will always be a yearning for just a bit of that secure and satisfying feeling that the past can evoke.

Let's hope that once in a while we all spend some time in the ballroom. ●

Christmas Goodies

Rosalie Bader, BSP

I graduated with a bachelor of science in pharmacy in 1966 from the University of Saskatchewan in Saskatoon. I retired from pharmacy last year after working as a community pharmacist for 21 years with Canada Safeway Limited, but my first job after graduation was as a hospital pharmacist at the Grey Nuns Hospital in Regina, Saskatchewan, the province's capital city. The hospital later became Pasqua Hospital, which it remains. This story took place while I was working there.

The pharmacy dispensary was located on the main floor, with an office and library across the hall. The manufacturing room, which every hospital pharmacy had, was located one floor below in the basement, and lots of items were prepared there to be used as ward stock. We made gallons of Savlon solutions of three different strengths and gallons of denatured alcohol, which was 70 percent alcohol with methylene blue added. We made skin lotion with benzaldehyde added to give it a pleasant almond scent. Some of the lotion was tinted blue and some pink and put into small bottles to be sent to the maternity ward for the new mothers. We also produced menthol ointment, a preparation similar to Desitin ointment, and various other skin preparations.

One Christmas, we decided we would like to make something special for the staff on the wards. We came up with the idea of making chocolate suppositories. We had one suppository mold that would make only six suppositories at a time, so we borrowed another mold from the other hospital in the city. We purchased milk chocolate bars and went into production.

It took several attempts with the addition of some paraffin wax to get perfect chocolate suppositories. We then wrapped each one in red or green foil. We also decorated sliding powder boxes with red and green foil and labeled them with the ward numbers. We put the suppositories into the boxes and proudly delivered them to the nursing stations with our best wishes for the Christmas season.

We were anxious to see how they would be received. Our efforts were appreciated, but somehow the nurses didn't want to eat them. They didn't want to believe that they were pure chocolate and suggested we had laced them with Ex-Lax! Oh well, it's the thought that counts. ●

All in a Day's Work

Rosalie Bader, BSP

It was the weekend before Christmas, and it was my turn to work in the hospital's pharmacy. That meant working alone on Friday evening until 9 pm and 8-hour days on Saturday and Sunday. The pharmacy was located on the first floor of the hospital. On the same wing was EENT (eye, ear, nose, and throat), which had been emptied of patients for the Christmas break.

The hallway into which the pharmacy wicket opened was dark. It was 8:45 pm on Friday, and I was preparing to close up when suddenly a man jumped at me through the open wicket. Over his head he had a white bag with eye openings cut out, and he was holding a weapon. He pointed the weapon at me and demanded drugs, giving names I didn't understand.

Trying not to show the panic I felt, I asked him to repeat what he had said. My voice came out in a higher pitch than normal. He repeated several names, one of which was "coke," and added, "Be quiet, or I will hit you." Had I already locked the safe, my hands would have been too shaky to work the combination to open it. However, it was still open, so I went to it and began to hand him boxes of injectable narcotics.

As suddenly as he had come, he dropped the boxes, turned to run, and jumped back out through the wicket. I think there was an accomplice in the hallway who had signaled to him. I immediately called the hospital switchboard to tell them I had been robbed. I then proceeded to do a narcotics count and determined that nothing was missing.

In no time, the police arrived and began to do some fingerprinting. They also had to take my prints because I had, without thinking, picked up some of the boxes that were left behind on the counter. Then, I had to go to the police station and look at mug shots to see whether I could make an identification of the robber.

While I was at the police station, I was sneezing and had watery eyes and a runny nose. I am prone to seasonal allergies, but this episode was the first time an allergic reaction had been triggered by an emotional response.

I learned the next day that at the same time I was robbed, security was called to one of the wards because a patient had grabbed one of the dietary aides and pulled her onto the bed with him. I also found out that on the afternoon of the attempted robbery an unknown man had been at the pharmacy asking what time we closed and that the pharmacist who had talked to him remarked that this seemed kind of strange. It was also discovered later that I had missed counting one strength of morphine injection and that we were one box short.

I continued to work the rest of the weekend on my own. Several times during the day, a hospital staff worker stopped at the wicket and said, "This is a stickup! Ha ha!"

The following Monday, bars were installed across the wicket. ●

An Unlikely Santa

Andrea S. Franks, PharmD, BCPS

Mr. Smith was a regular patient in our interdisciplinary geriatric clinic. He was a lifelong smoker who had advanced chronic obstructive pulmonary disease and hypertension. He did not have much money and had difficulty affording his complex medication regimen. He also had trouble understanding the regimen. Caring for Mr. Smith required a great deal of time and attention.

After several years of care in our clinic, he was finally on an affordable, streamlined medication regimen. With our assistance, he successfully quit smoking. On a cold, gray December morning, several months after our clinic closed, my doorbell rang. I was surprised to find Mr. Smith standing on my front porch, looking a bit like a scruffy Santa, loaded down with stuffed animals, watches, and other Christmas gifts for my children. He even had something for me—a Shoney's gift certificate. He said, "Use that to buy your old man a steak."

I wondered why he was being so generous. And then, I remembered something he told us when he left the clinic one day: "I look forward to coming to my appointments because I can tell that you really care about me. I feel like you are my family." ●

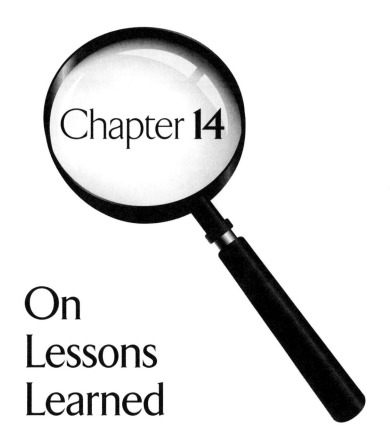

Chapter **14**

On
Lessons
Learned

Wherever the art of medicine is loved,
there also is love of humanity.

—**Hippocrates**

Lessons from Palermo

Heather J. Johnson, PharmD, BCPS

A small mention of "a potential international opportunity" probably piqued my interest as I set out to apply for my first position after postgraduate residency training. In fact, I still have the job posting in my files. I could not have imagined then the adventures and opportunities that would unfold upon taking that job, which included teaching a group of Italian nurses about transplant medications.

Teaching Italian nurses about immunosuppressive medications via a translator was surprisingly rewarding. Although they spoke very little English and I knew no Italian at the time, I could generally understand the questions they asked. They were the same questions I had been asked by any number of English-speaking nurses before. Teaching nurses stateside soon evolved into developing pharmacy services, both clinical and distributive, in Italy. Although I felt I had sufficient experience in providing these services, I soon learned there was a world of pharmacy I knew nothing about.

Any pharmacist who has traveled has walked into a foreign pharmacy just to check things out and usually will marvel at the medications that can be purchased without a prescription. However, these cursory tours tell us very little about differences in the operation of pharmacy, the provision of medication therapy, and the cultural attitudes toward medications and even pharmacists. Little in my pharmacy education had prepared me specifically for these challenges, but I came to know just how well prepared I was in the coming months and learned some lessons along the way.

Lesson 1: Communication
"Is there a periodic table in the pharmacy?" Translation: I would like to give 20 mEq of potassium chloride, but the tablets are labeled 600 mg.

Be clear, and ask for clarification. When asking a question, know what endpoint you are seeking. When giving a response, understand what problem needs to be solved.

Lesson 2: Calculation

"What is the volume of a sphere?" Translation: A surgeon wants a reasonable idea of what volume might be drained from a cyst of 10 cm diameter.

When presented with seemingly bizarre questions, be flattered that you or any pharmacist can be part of the solution. Know that your unique educational background and knowledge of resources will enable you to solve problems as they present themselves. After all, people will not ask you the questions to which they can easily find the answers.

Lesson 3: Context

"That sounds like something I use to deworm my horses." Translation: *Strongyloides stercoralis* is more common in Italy than in the United States.

Don't assume that the environment is universal. Take time to learn about the uniqueness of any setting or location as you begin to solve problems.

Lesson 4: Creativity

"I want it now" versus "You don't always get what you want." Translation: A request for 15 L of 5% sodium chloride, not commercially available.

When the obvious solution (pun unintended) is not available, your ability to think outside the box and explore other possibilities and potential solutions will enable you to provide what the patient and provider need.

Lesson 5: Health Care

"It looks like you are overdue for a tetanus shot." Translation: You are going to get a tetanus shot.

If we are fortunate, we don't have to navigate or interface with many aspects of our own health care system. This ignorance, however, puts us at a disadvantage in helping our patients who necessarily must navigate a sometimes complex and daunting system.

While in Italy, I asked very basic questions about how the system functioned and in doing so learned more about two systems than I had known previously. I also received a few lessons in what can be done very well in other systems. I accompanied my husband to the local health office to obtain his vaccination records. Before providing him with a copy of the record, the nurse noted that he was overdue for a tetanus booster. So he got his updated records, booster included!

I was fortunate to have experienced the birth of two healthy babies during my time in Palermo. A labor and delivery nurse asked me how much it would cost to have a baby in the United States, as she had heard it was very expensive. Being a first-time mother, I didn't know. However, I knew it was more than the cost in

Italy, which the nurse assured me in a public hospital was free for any woman. In fact, I shared a room with women from all walks of Italian life and their newborns.

As a health care professional, I learned a lot from these experiences. I now feel more empowered to navigate many aspects of the U.S. system that I probably was ignorant of before, and I believe I can explain some of the advantages and disadvantages of another system.

Lesson 6: Understanding

"*Straniera.*" Translation: Stranger, or foreigner.

In many ways, our patients are strangers in a foreign land. We often speak a "medical" language in front of patients and their families, which is foreign to many of them. Having been the foreigner has helped me become a better pharmacist, and all pharmacists can use their own experiences of fear and lack of understanding to help patients in similar situations.

Although not all pharmacists or pharmacy students have or desire the types of opportunities I have had, I believe there is great value in providing international educational experiences for pharmacy students. I have been able, through my continued relationships with Italian pharmacists, to facilitate advanced pharmacy practice elective experiences for a handful of students. Upon exit interviews, the recurring themes of self-awareness, communication, and empathy are evident, and I know these lessons will last these young pharmacists (and myself) a lifetime. ●

What's in a Name?

Mary Shue, RPh

In the early 1980s, when we were first learning about AIDS and feeling a little nervous about interacting with AIDS patients, I was working in a university health service setting. Our first patient that we knew had HIV was "Fred." I'm not even sure if AIDS had been referred to as HIV at that point, and, for sure, no medicines to treat it were on the market yet. Fred was just as cranky as he could be every time he came into the pharmacy.

Finally, one day, I decided to start greeting him by name when he arrived at the window. That changed everything. His whole demeanor softened every time we would greet him with, "Fred, how's it going today?" We heard that he had died in another state not too long after.

Since then, I have never underestimated the power of simply calling a person by his or her name. ●

House Calls

Sarah T. Melton, PharmD, BCPP, CGP

Do you remember when physicians used to make house calls? Very few providers can afford to offer this type of care any longer, but I have found that making house calls with my students is much more than a valuable learning experience.

Miss Virginia is 92 years young and lives close to the clinic, but she does not drive and hates to be dependent on anyone for transportation. She called one day saying that she was having a terrible reaction to her clonidine patch. Miss Virginia had uncontrolled isolated systolic hypertension and had been through many trials of medications, the patch being her most recent. When we arrived at her house, she had refreshments waiting for us. My students took her blood pressure (still uncontrolled), and I looked at her reaction, which resembled a first-degree burn. We changed her medication to a calcium channel blocker and continued to make weekly visits to her home to check on her. When she needed labs, my students would pick her up, bring her to the clinic, and take care of her every step of the way. I believe that the combination of love, attention, and diltiazem finally got her blood pressure under control.

When you see patients in the clinic, you can only picture their living situation in your head, and the picture depends solely on what they tell you. Nothing compares to a firsthand look in the home. Mr. Johnson, a beloved figure in the community, was a retired school teacher and baseball coach. He had developed significant dementia that was rapidly progressing. It took his wife 2 to 3 hours to prepare him for a clinic visit, and when he was there, he was uncommunicative, except to ask repeatedly when he could go home. She told me how terrible the behavioral problems were and that the family was getting no rest. When my students and I visited the home, Mr. Johnson constantly paced, and we saw the path worn in the carpet. We saw the broken furniture that he had thrown the night before when he was psychotic, thinking he was back in the war. We saw him change clothes three times in the half-hour we were there. We saw the effects of dementia on the family. He continually asked, "When can I go home?"

Miss Polly is 72 years old and complains constantly of pain and being cold. She often runs short with her hydrocodone, so I wondered whether family members could be taking it. She lives in a small house with five other people, and the odor and fog of cigarette smoke are nauseating. She sleeps in a hospital bed in a bedroom with her niece. In the middle of July, she was in the bed wrapped in winter pajamas, heavy socks, and at least three heavy blankets tucked around her. She would get out of bed only to use the restroom. When I asked to see her medications, she reached under her pillow and brought out her purse. She told me she always keeps her medicine on her person or under her pillow as she sleeps, so now I saw that it was more likely that Miss Polly was taking more hydrocodone than prescribed because it would be like robbing a bank to get to the medicine.

My students and I recently made a visit to see a patient with a hemoglobin A1c of 10 who needed a new glucometer. All the questions we asked in the clinic about diet and exercise were answered with somewhat acceptable answers. Interestingly, the answers in the clinic were not consistent with what we saw in the home. As we entered the kitchen, we saw bologna sandwiches, Little Debbie Swiss Cake Rolls, and 16-oz bottles of Mountain Dew. It was time for more intervention rather than a new glucometer!

I can tell numerous other stories about how medications are stored, strange medication administration rituals, and the effects of illness on the family. The main lesson I have learned from visiting patients at home is that the assumptions you make during a clinic visit are often altered. It almost always changes the intervention and education you provide—for the better. ●

Life Lessons

Sharon Connor, PharmD

I had just completed my second year of pharmacy school and had the opportunity to participate in a month-long medical mission to the Dominican Republic offered through Creighton University and the Institute for Latin American Concern. I did not yet have much pharmacy knowledge, but I went into the experience with enthusiasm and armed with as many references as I could drag along with me.

To get to our clinic location, we rode in the back of a pickup truck to our drop-off point and then hiked the remaining 4 hours. The tiny village was inaccessible by road; the main modes of transportation were by donkey or on foot.

The clinic was to be set up in a run-down barn in the mountainous village. The exam rooms were separated by sheets hanging from ropes. We prepared the clinic each day by walking 15 minutes up the road with gallon water jugs in hand to the river, our water source. We needed water to wash our hands.

On the first day, a line of more than 50 people formed. The first patient was a young child who had a horrible skin infection, with wounds that were weeping. After the exam, the attending physician approached me in my "pharmacy" (a small supply of medications organized on stacked slats of wood) and said, "It looks like the patient has impetigo, what do you think we should give him?"

I stared back, a bit shocked, and thought to myself, "You are the attending; you have all of the knowledge." I said to him, "I am not sure," and deferred to him.

He immediately replied, "Oh no, this is a team effort, we are all in a new and strange setting. You are the expert on the drug supply and medication choices, and I want you to help determine the appropriate treatment." I consulted my multiple references and came up with an answer. We all agreed.

I stayed with a Dominican family during the mission. They had 11 children, but they gave me the best room in the three-room thatched-roof house, which consisted of a bedroom, a "family room," and a kitchen. They did not have electricity or running water. The water supply for the house was the river, which was visited many times a day by the 7-, 9-, and 10-year-old girls, who carried five-gallon tin cans. Even with their hardships, all the members of the family were so giving. Their biggest concern was to tend to me and to make sure that I was happy. Even though our clinic group ate meals together, my "mother" prepared a second dinner for me each night when I returned home.

Toward the end of my stay, the children asked me to ask their mother if they could go on a hiking expedition to the "big cave." I was by no means fluent in Spanish, but facial expressions and body language go a long way. After I asked their mother, in my broken Spanish, if the children could go with me, she looked at them with that look that mothers give their children when they have knowingly done something wrong. She then smiled at me and said, "Not this time." After thinking about it, I finally figured out what their mother already knew; it was a ploy to get out of doing chores. I thought to myself, "These children have so much spirit; they are so happy and mischievous." Even though we speak different languages and are from different cultures, we really are all the same. Children around the world are looking for ways to have fun and just be children.

This experience has molded me to be the person I am today. I thought I was going on a mission to help people; little did I know that I would receive so much in return. All people have much to offer and teach us. Not only did I learn a lot about my role as a pharmacist in a health care team, I learned even more about how to live my life. ●

Understanding Everyone

Kathleen J. Cross, PharmD

I was a new pharmacist in a retail setting. One afternoon, a woman came to the pharmacy to pick up her antibiotics. During pharmacy school, we were taught the importance of taking antibiotics until they were all gone because "the bugs get smart" and the patient's infection could worsen if the patient stopped taking the medication too soon. So, in counseling this woman, I told her to take all her medication because "the bugs get smart." She shrieked, "I've got bugs?"

Well, of course, I learned a very valuable lesson that day. As a pharmacist, I have to know my audience. I have to consider each patient's knowledge level and relate to the patient in a manner that he or she can understand. I have to have compassion for patients' feelings and understand that they are not always at their best when needing medical care and don't need anything else to stress them out.

After a few years, I went back to school and obtained my PharmD, completed a residency, and moved to the hospital setting. Although it has been almost 6 years, I still run into old customers from the retail pharmacy, and they greet me with hugs and well wishes. I love my new job, but I sure miss making people feel good about coming to a retail pharmacy where someone genuinely cares about their health care. ●

Feeding the Monkey: A Pharmacist's Leader-Development Lesson Learned

W. Mike Heath, RPh, MBA

Today, leadership in the pharmacy profession is of critical importance as a key component to the future success of both the profession and the practice of pharmacy.

During my career as a pharmacist and commissioned officer in the U.S. Army, I learned firsthand about leadership and leader development. Some of what I learned was through formalized programs of study. The vast majority of what I learned about leadership as both a pharmacist and an officer, however, was a direct result of on-the-job experiences in a variety of assignments.

When I was a major, I was assigned to Fort Sill, Oklahoma, as chief (director) of pharmacy of Reynolds Army Community Hospital. My organizational chain-of-command reporting structure was through the chief administrative officer, or, as it was termed in the Army, deputy commander for administration, who was my immediate boss.

As it turned out, my boss was a tall, red-headed senior officer from rural Arkansas, with a quintessential Southern accent. He was a colorful individual who called it as he saw it, but most importantly, he understood leadership and the importance of leader development, especially with the junior officers for whom he was responsible. Bottom line: He was a great mentor and role model.

One of my most memorable experiences in pharmacy leader development resulted from an appointment with my boss. I do not recall the specific issue, but I felt the need to seek his guidance on a problem I was dealing with in my department. In communicating the issue, I may have come across as complaining or uncertain. Before I could finish explaining, he stopped me in my tracks and said, "Don't bring me that monkey to feed."

I did not have a clue what he meant, so I responded, "Sir, I don't know what you are talking about."

He replied, "Mike, what I mean is don't bring a problem to me and dump it at my doorstep. If you come to talk about a problem, I also expect you to be prepared to discuss potential solutions."

That mentoring encounter stuck with me for my entire 30-year career in the military, and as I became more senior in rank and committed to mentor and develop the next generation of Army pharmacy officers, I often shared my early leader-development experience of "Don't bring me that monkey to feed." ●

A Question of Age

Keith Patterson, PharmD

I worked on a busy pain management team and had a lot of patient contact with very sick people. I walked into a patient's room and discussed his pain level and his current treatment. I then said to the person sitting at the bedside, "Do you have any questions about your father's treatment?"

He responded, "Oh, he's my younger brother."

The man in the bed was so sick he looked like an elderly man, not the younger brother of the person sitting next to him. I now know not to assume anything about a patient or his or her family. If others are in the room, I ask if they're related and, if so, in what way. •

No Thanks

David K. Records, BPharm

I was working in a busy, suburban retail pharmacy when an elderly gentleman wearing overalls presented me with a prescription for an erectile dysfunction drug. Even though he wasn't familiar to me, he did have a profile on our computer. As the technician entered the prescription, an interaction message noting the man's nitroglycerin flashed on the screen. We stopped, and I called his doctor, who reinforced my decision not to fill the prescription. When the patient came back to the pharmacy, I told him about the interaction, that it could be potentially fatal, and that we wouldn't be filling the prescription. He looked at me with complete irritation and said, "You're just tryin' to spoil my fun!" and stormed out of the store.

Although I had potentially saved the gentleman's life, he was not the least bit grateful, and I never saw him again in the pharmacy. However, being a professional means that despite the consequences, such as angering—or even losing—a patient, your patients' well-being is your first priority. I have been thanked by many other patients, and that certainly is more pleasant and affirming. This situation spoke to me about how doing the right thing as a professional pharmacist is not always popular, but it is necessary. ●

Martin

Pamela Stewart-Kuhn, RPh, MPA, CGP

He is an intimidating figure, built like a linebacker. At about 6′4″ and 250-plus pounds, I wouldn't want to meet him on a dark street at night. He's got a big, booming baritone voice with a Southern drawl and a wicked sense of humor. He's loud—very loud. I wasn't sure what to think when he first came to my pharmacy window with his elderly mom, a military widow. "Take the rest of the day off y'all!" he would come in and tell us. I came to learn that he is actually an 8-year-old child trapped in a 45-year-old body. He's also the biggest Auburn football fan in "L.A." (lower Alabama).

As a mom, pregnant twice in my 30s, I always thought that having a child with a disability would be the worst possible outcome. I was blessed with two healthy children. However, Martin has allowed me a glimpse into another world. I've realized that "different" doesn't have to mean "terrible." I've never asked about the nature of his disability. I actually don't think of him as disabled, and I don't think he considers himself any different from the rest of us. He's simply Martin, the big kid in the bright orange Auburn T-shirt. ●

A Different Way of Seeing

Nancy Brady Smith, RPh, CDM-Diabetes

Ancora imparo means "I am still learning" and is attributed to the 87-year-old Michelangelo. Like him, I am still learning and have found that nearly every pharmacist has been able to teach me something. That's one of the great advantages to working with so many people over the years. The mentoring process is ongoing and perhaps even subtle at times. Often, we learn to do something a better, easier way. Sometimes it's a new technique, or it's a more effective way to communicate with the patients we serve. At times, we even learn how best *not* to do something.

Once, the lesson I learned was how to be more compassionate. Lori was a technician I hired many years ago. She had a gap of nearly 5 years in her work history, and I wondered whether she would be dependable. From her interview, I found out that she was a mother of two young boys and was just reentering the workforce. Although she was on welfare, she had plans to go back to school to finish her education.

At the time, I wondered if I would be taking a gamble by hiring her. In the end, I decided to give her a try, and, boy, did that gamble pay off! She was extremely dependable, had a great work ethic, and was upbeat about everything. In her words, she was "blessed" despite the difficulties of rearing two boys, returning to school full time, working, and being on welfare. I worked with her for several years until she graduated as a nurse.

One day when we were working together, a patient on welfare came in to pick up a prescription. The prescription was written for Phospho-soda, which is an over-the-counter (OTC) medication. In the state in which I reside, OTC medications are not, for the most part, covered by Medicaid; however, prescription medications are. Thus, even if the patient has a prescription for an OTC medication, she would have to pay for it. Most patients on Medicaid cannot afford to pay for any medication that isn't covered by their insurance, no matter how inexpensive.

In this patient's case, this medication, being used for a procedure, was medically necessary, yet the patient did not have the money to pay for it. At that, Lori said that she would pay for it, and she did. She, who could ill afford it herself, paid for the patient's prescription.

I admit that I was embarrassed by my lack of generosity and compassion. That I, who could easily afford it, couldn't see that the patient's need outweighed the cost, but Lori did.

Whether she knows it or not, that act of stewardship has forever changed the way I look at patients and their needs. I believe I have become a more caring pharmacist and have at times done the same thing for others—whether it's a college student away from home and out of cash, a person who just can't afford a needed antibiotic, or some other equally important reason. No, I don't pay for everyone's prescriptions, and I don't do it all the time, but sometimes it is as Lori said, "Well, she needs it, doesn't she?" ●